CONVERSATION
WITH
THE HEALER

---

*The Herbs are for the Healing
of the Nations*

Recorded by A.V.

Table of Contents

Genesis   The Account of Creation 1

Chapter 1   The Truth About History 7

Chapter 2   Why Do People Get Sick? 20

Chapter 3   Natural, Unnatural and the Supernatural 30

Chapter 4   The Conversation 42

Chapter 5   The Interview 55

Chapter 6   Electric Food for the Electric Body 78

GOD's Recommended Medicine 123

GOD's Creations 135

Acknowledgments 137

Index 139

Note to Readers

I am the recorder of this wisdom.
This knowledge is not mine.
But it is my responsibility to share.
I'm only the messenger.

The Great Awakening.

-A.V.

Conversation with the Healer

GENESIS

The Account of Creation

In the beginning, God created the heavens and the earth. The earth was empty, a formless mass cloaked in darkness. And the **Spirit of God** was hovering over its surface Then God said, "Let there be light," and there was light. And God saw that it was good. Then he separated the **light from the darkness.** God called the light "day" and the darkness "night". Together these made up one day.

And God said, "Let there be space between the waters, to separate water from water." And so it was. God made this space to separate the waters above from the waters below. And God called the space "sky". This happened on the second day.

And God said, "Let the waters beneath the sky be gathered into one place so dry ground may appear." And so it was. God named the dry ground "land" and the water "seas." And God saw that it was good. Then God said, "Let the land burst forth with every sort of grass and seed-bearing plant. And let there be seed-bearing fruit trees. The seeds will then produce the kind of plants and trees from which they came." And so it was. The land was filled with seed-bearing plants and trees, and their seeds produced plants and trees of like kind. And God saw that it was good. This all happened on the third day.

And God said, "Let bright lights appear in the sky to separate the day from the night. They will be signs to mark off the seasons, the days, and the years. Let their light shine down upon the earth." And so it was. For God made two great lights, the sun, and the moon, to shine down upon the earth. The greater one, **the sun,** presides during the day; the lesser one, **the moon,** presides through the night. He also made **the stars.** God set these lights in the heavens to light the earth, to govern the day and the night, and to separate the light from the darkness. And God saw that it was good. This all happened on the fourth day.

And God said, "Let the waters swarm with fish and other life. Let the skies be filled with birds of every kind." So God created great sea creatures and every sort of fish and every kind of bird. And God saw that it was good. Then God blessed them, saying, "Let the fish multiply and fill the oceans. Let the birds increase and fill the earth." This all happened on the fifth day.

And God said, "Let the earth bring forth every kind of animal--livestock, small animals, and wildlife." And so it was. God made all sorts of wild animals, livestock, and small animals, each able to reproduce more of its kind. And God saw that it was good.

Then God said, "**Let us make people**" in our image, be like ourselves. They will be masters over all life—the fish in the sea, the birds in the sky, and all the livestock, wild animals, "and small animals." So God created people in his image; God patterned them after himself; male and female he created them.

God blessed them and told them, "Multiply and fill the earth and subdue it. Be masters over the fish and birds and all the animals." And God said, "Look! I have given you the seed-bearing plants throughout the earth and all the fruit trees for your food. And I have given all the grasses and other green plants to the animals and birds for their food." And so it was. Then God looked over all he had made and he saw that it was excellent in every way. This all happened on the sixth day.

The creation of the **heavens** and the **earth** and everything in them was completed. On the seventh day, having finished his task, God rested from all his work. **God blessed the seventh day and declared it holy** because it was the day when he rested from his work of creation. This is the account of the creation of heaven and earth.

Revelation 22:2

Through the middle of the street of the city, also, on either side of the river, the tree of life with its twelve kinds of fruit, yielding its fruit each month. The leaves of the tree were for the healing of the nations.

Genesis 1:29

And God said, "Behold, I have given you every plant yielding seed that is on the face of all the earth, and every tree with seed in its fruit. You shall have them for food.

Ezekiel 47:12

And on the banks, on both sides of the river, there will grow all kinds of trees for food. Their leaves will not wither, nor their fruit fails, but they will bear fresh fruit every month because the water for them flows from the sanctuary. Their fruit will be for food, and their leaves for healing."

Proverbs 15:17

Better is a dinner of herbs where love is, than a fattened ox and hatred with it.

Chapter 1

The Truth About History

H. Welcome! Today we're going to attempt to peel off layers of historical occurrences. We, as African people, have been told many things by many people about our history. But we have not done the proper historical documentation that is needed in the area of nutrition. We have done the history of different Empires. About the **Kings and Queens** that we never needed and DON'T NEED NOW! But I have yet to hear about our work that was dedicated to healing.

Why is it so important? Well, as we go into this thing called healing. History again becomes the vehicle that we're going to use to travel towards that goal that we're looking for.

We are looking for a goal because **we're sick.** Something we didn't have in our environment. So, healing and entertaining the subject one has to remember that it has to be tied to the cosmic procession. **Healing has to be consistent with life itself.** If it isn't, then it's not healing. The component has to be from life. So, going into this journey, back into the past to find what was it that was happening in Africa. What was occurring?

We can begin with that Black woman, "Mama!" You know the Black woman that many countries identified as being a savage. When they first saw her without any clothes. Everybody was amazed! The lady was naked! Not that she's natural. She was naked! **But she didn't know that she was naked.** That's the way she was since creation, the natural way to be. But the foreigner saw her as a savage and many of us, her children, also collaborated. We think that it is correct the way that we view her. And we, her children also said that she was a savage.

The Ph.D. professor with his suit and tie. When he stole, that's when his beginning started with the Black woman without any clothes.

"It's embarrassing!" It's what the professor said to us. **Shame takes over.** I am ashamed of my history. Because it began with a naked woman in the forest of Africa. But that naked woman was more than just the image you saw in your eyes that was running around crazy. She was saying that we can live without any clothes. My Mama can live without any clothes in the forest of Africa. She could walk around and no one was jumping on her. Well, was she a savage? Or was she showing that she lives in a highly ethical and moral society?

I had a conversation in Brazil where a Russian said "Ay, before you say something about your people, just remember that your Mama didn't have any clothes on just 500 years ago."

But I said "Why did you stop there? Without no clothes?"

"What do you mean?" Said the Russian.

You're saying my Mama had no clothes 500 years ago. And she didn't have any supermarkets. She didn't have any doctors and hospitals. she didn't have any disease. Mama didn't have clothes, alcohol, drugs, or money and by the way, we are going to go into it a little bit more.

Do you see what's happening? Everything that's occurring today in the 20th century. **We're misinterpreted.** The Black race have been vulnerable to the research that others have done about our Mama. But as we look closer, we find that Mama was ethical, shameless, and moral. I wish that we can do this now. So, we can't think that she's a savage. Tell your woman today to walk the streets without no clothes on and see who is the savage? As we leave that part of Mama where she shows that she was highly ethical and that she lives in a beautiful environment with her brothers and sisters.

Now we go to her diet, that's very important! Because you see her diet, it was consistent with her cellular predisposition. Her diet was like the eagle.

The eagle doesn't eat the diet of the Kitkat bird. Because the Kitkat bird only eats fruits and seeds. But when you go to the eagle which is a bird, he eats meat. Then we leave that bird and we go to the gorilla and the polar bear-like I like to use.

The polar bear has to kill his food. The polar bear eats blood, not so for the gorilla. The gorilla has nothing to do with blood, he eats leaves. The gorilla doesn't have to kill his food, his food is all around him.

So, the question I'm getting to is this: Gorilla has his food designed by nature. The eagle has his food designed by nature or GOD. Do you believe that we are exempt? No, we're not! We have to follow that same law that rules that cosmic arrangement. The one that dictates, not the ones that are philosophy. The one that dictates from the core of life since creation. We are subject to that same law.

There's a little frog in Puerto Rico they call the Coqui. If any of you have visited Puerto Rico you will hear that little frog all night singing "Co-kee!, Co-kee! Co-kee!" If you move that frog from that island of Puerto Rico and put it 7km away, the frog dies. The frog will die, the frog will no longer sing. We're seeing that this frog has to live in that cosmic arrangement to survive and to live at its optimum level of life and expression.

Well, are we exempt? Our Mothers didn't have any rice, beans, hog maw, or chitterlings. Our Mother didn't eat garbage and she didn't produce garbage. She didn't have ham because she didn't eat meat. This is interesting, our Mother didn't eat meat? NO! There was no cow in Africa. They didn't have chicken, ham, or goat. Those things aren't African. But there are many Africans today that believe that yam is African.

Is Cassava African? When an African believes that these things are African or natural. Well, it only means that we have to go and do further research that's all.

Something has been derailed. So, when you believe that starches such as yam were part of your diet well, that slavery is back again or never left.

So our Mother, living in an alkaline environment didn't eat the things that will bring disease. This is why she showed that she didn't need hospitals. There's something else about this Black Woman in the jungle of Africa. She didn't have any disobedient children. There was no chaos, there was peace.

I, unlike most of my brothers and sisters who have been to Egypt. They researched King Ramsey, Nefertiti, Cleopatra. I was never interested in Egyptian history. No, NEVER! Maybe just to know that it has occurred. Not that I was interested to extrapolate from Egypt any substance that would support and enhance my life. No! Egypt does not have any of those components. But I can travel a little bit west from Egypt and go into the jungle of Africa. Yah, the jungle where my Mama lived. In that environment, I can find a plant known as Concansa. Which if you were 90 or 100 years of age and you find yourself at a deficit sexually. You only have to take Concansa once and you have renewed again. That you get out of the jungle.

We stay in the jungle and there's another one called "See-ha." It's a plant that Michael Jackson's son had the opportunity to receive the benefit from. He had a tumor in his frontal lobe and he sneezed that out in twenty minutes. That herb is another jungle herb.

Then we go a little to the south of Guinea and we find Namibia. Namibia has another plant known as the Hoodia. This is a plant that upon ingesting it, you will not eat for days. Because it is nourishing every cell in your body. Then we go to the Tabernanthe Iboga, the Great Iboga. The plant relaxes the body and places the body in a state of bliss. There can't be any emotional problems after ingesting this plant.

But those of you come back with souvenirs. You came back with souvenirs from the jungle. I came back with healing. Because somewhere in my little journey on this planet I heard something from my parents, that I was obedient. My mother and my Grandmother never had any complaints from the neighbor or the community that I did something to offend them. No, I didn't indulge in that. So somewhere in my conversation with my Grandmother and Mama, they would share with me this.

I heard something like "Be obedient." To be obedient is a very necessary thing especially now. When GOD placed us in the forest of Africa. He placed with us a mandate and our food, that's all we needed. But today I have been taken away from that natural cosmic arrangement.

"I need a guru, I need a preacher, I need a leader," that is only showing us we are confused. **We need help, we are sick.**

So, in peeling off the layers of history and excavating further. We found that Mama was far from being a savage. She was the one that was in direct compliance with the arrangement of life. It was because of her that I can be the servant that I am to you.

Yes, I enjoy my position and I should enjoy it. I've enjoyed every position I occupied. I like everything.

I love everything. So as a servant to you. I'm only letting you know that the accomplishment that I have been accredited with, belongs to that naked woman in the forest of Africa.

I'm not asking the Black race to take their clothes off. No! Wish we could though because it would be the optimal level in expression and living life. Because the cells in the body would breathe. Today we cover up all ourselves. This is why when someone takes their clothes off, under those clothes look a little bit more worn out than the face and the arm. Why? They have been deprived of oxygen for maybe 50 or 60 years.

Mama didn't have that! Mama didn't tax daddy.

"Hey you, you have to buy me this dress that I saw. You have to buy me the Louis Vuitton shoes."

Mama didn't need shoes. She walked as GOD made her. She was in direct compliance with GOD.

But today, her son was taken away from her 500 years ago. We no longer live by the dictates of that woman. I eat chicken, hog, rice, and beans. At the end of that, I find myself at a deficit. I was sick at 30. I was impotent from 27 on to 30. Asthmatic from birth.

A baby is being born sick? Yes! I'm one of those babies, born sick. That is against life procession, a sick baby. A baby should be born healthy. But to clear that and to bring it to light that we can understand. When babies were born healthy. The quality of the sperm that made babies 500 years ago in the jungle of Africa. That sperm was not impregnated with hog, rice, beans, or potato. That sperm was of a different quality, it was an alkaline sperm. Why? Because Mommy and Daddy only ate what was alkaline food, that's all nature makes. Nature doesn't produce an acid substance. Nature can only produce alkaline substances.

We're going back to Mama again. We have to travel to and from because every time we visit her, we see we're in the deficit and we are all going deeper. We should stop it! This is where nature comes in, the sperm that makes the baby, that made the babies didn't need to be born in a hospital. Mama had her baby under a tree. Mama didn't need a doctor, that's a violation when you need a doctor. YOU have been violated for 500 years. Mama wasn't violated, she lives by the laws of life. So, her baby could be born under a tree and the baby would be born healthy. Because the quality of the sperm was what GOD would like all of us to be or to produce or to inject into a woman or to offer. The quality of the sperm was alkaline.

Today, not so. Because we have been severed from Mama and eating all of the things we're consuming today. The quality of our sperm is very much acid. Babies are being born autistic, with diabetes and cancer.

Ladies and gentlemen, brothers and sisters... something is wrong isn't it? And what is wrong? We were taken away from our natural rhythm from that organic environment. Our babies are being born sick and I am one of those babies. But when I began to research Mama and my diet and begin to change with the help of a Mexican. Now I'm 80 years of age and I have a little girl, she's two!

That is showing me that just revisiting Mama a little bit. I was able to accomplish something I thought was not possible. So, let us not lose focus. The environment that Mama lived within afforded her peace. This is what we are trying to bring to you. An alkaline substance.

Because when your brother in 1988 proved to the Supreme Court of New York and the world.

"Yes, we cured AIDS, we cured diabetes, we cured!"

We should not be afraid to claim it. Like my sister said, "That I didn't know the Black race has been accredited with the cure of diseases."

When she said that, it resonated well with me. Because it is the truth. If this is true, what prevents our so-called "leaders" from supporting this entity? We need healing, all of us need healing. What's preventing them? The same things that prevented my brother from recognizing what I had offered him. He passed away 25 years ago and he was a preacher. I am not a preacher! I am a servant to my community.

I wanted to be a musician. I wanted to be like John Coltrane. I wanted to be like Pharoah Sanders. But no! Nature said shut your mouth! This is what you have been designed for! But in that design that I recognize. I find myself in the middle of it. The message I got is that I'm only the messenger of healing, I'm not the healer.

Yes, as I said we have reversed the reversible disease. But I am not the healer, the healer is a woman. Because healing needs a nurturer. Healing needs an understanding of nature and that's not a male. This is precisely why you will never see a cub following a daddy in the forest. Why? Daddy doesn't have the program of life embedded in his brain. It is Mama again! You will never see a cub following daddy. All males and females follow Mama, including that lion that the French man said "It's the king of the jungle." Well, if the lion is the king of the jungle. She must be something better than that! Because that lion came out of that lioness. But again, being severed from Mama, we take on this philosophical expression.

Yeah, that's where the breakdown begins. I cannot live by the dictate of that naked woman in the forest of Africa. I have to live by the dictate of the philosopher Socrates, Plato, Diogenes, and John Stuart Mill. All these people I'm supposed to know about why? I don't know. But I've been led there and my friends would use that against me. Because I haven't done any research in the area of philosophy. Because I'm not interested in philosophy, then or now. **I am interested in life.** Philosophy doesn't afford or offer any substance that you can add to the sequence or the arrangement of life. It doesn't offer that! But when you look at the jungle. Oh boy, you begin to see mushrooms and alkaline plants. Scientifically they are called phosphate, carbonate, iodide, bromide this what they are called scientifically.

That's all we had in the forest, PH levels of more than 7. What do I mean? That everything Mama ate in the forest of Africa had a PH level of more than 7. That means it's on the alkaline side. Today, I no longer eat anything less than 7 PH. I used to eat garlic which is 3.3 PH. I drank cow milk which is 6 or 5.5 PH. I ate meat. I ate starches that range in the 4s never anything that was 7 plus. I ate acid food and I get acid thoughts.

Mama! Yes, Tupac. You did a good job Tupac when you talked about Mama. Mama didn't have toilets. Mama didn't need toilets. I remember once, there was an argument between me and a professor from UCLA. This man was trying his endeavor best to show me that the Europeans have to be given credit for inventing the toilet.

I looked at him and said "I must be very wrong. I must be very mistaken."

Because this man is a professor at UCLA and he's telling me that the invention of the toilet was the greatest invention ever. Because I can flush my acid fecal matter into the ocean. Listen carefully now. He's trying to win an argument against me which I've never tried to win or lose. I cannot win or lose. I don't go into a debate or a dialogue to win. It is about understanding. I don't debate with anyone. I don't have to do that! But he said that because the Europeans invented the toilet, that he deserved much credit.

So, my response was this "My history shows that Mama didn't need a toilet. Because everything that she ate was alkaline. Because it was alkaline, it didn't leave any residue of poison or acid in her fecal matter. When it was broken down in her intestines by the villi. Mama can take her feces and put them in the ground and it should smell good."

With my little understanding and the little accomplishment that I have made over the 40 years of this particular giving. When I go to the toilet, I don't smell anything. But I remember when I couldn't stand it. I would have to spray the toilet. Sure! I had too! Because I was just like you. I'm a product of disease.

I asked my Mother "What was it that you and daddy were eating that helped to create the condition for me to be born with asthma?

She said "We used to eat conch, lobster, crab, shrimp."

Those are all scavengers. The scavengers are acid, very acid! My Mama and my daddy were eating crab, shrimp, conch, and lobster and they ate pork meat. So here they are, they were eating the scavengers. What category should we place Mama and daddy? If they were eating the scavengers. They are worse than the scavengers and I am the result of that diet. Then you tell me that I'm cool. Come on now, let's be cool. You know I'm sick. I have to be sick.

I'm lucky to have a child born to me at 78. I'm 80 now and my child is 2. That was because when I went to America and I met these people we called hippies. They were on the right path about diet. So, I was able to do something to make a change. Now, I could smile when I used to cry. I was placed in an insane asylum in New Jersey in 1961. The brother was schizophrenic and paranoid. To leave that state of paranoia and schizophrenia to now have patients come to us that are cured of schizophrenia and paranoia. Do you see what a diet does?

Mama again, the diet of Mama. Tupac I wish that you would have lived a little bit longer. I know you would have added something to the chapter. Because I like what you did with Mama. Mama is the basis of all life. It is Mama! So today we are bringing you this first chapter of this mother expression and offering this thing that we need today.

Because today I cannot love you. **How can I love you when I don't even love myself?** I'll blow my brain out! I take pills to take me away because everything is ugly. We didn't have those things occurring in the jungle. It was very peaceful, it was harmonious. There wasn't violence, there couldn't be violence. Because they ate alkaline foods. That's all they ate! In my research, I find that the people that were brought to us that were insane. Well, we just changed their diet, took their clothes off, and immediately they calmed down and they slept that night. Why? Because **the brain was not invaded with uric acid or carbonic acid.** NO! Mama did not have that in her diet.

So yes, this is the first chapter. A first of a series of lectures that we will bring to you in helping us to see that Mama was not a savage. She was in direct compliance with the energy of life and that she didn't need a Guru or the Preacher or the Dalai Lama. She didn't need any of those people. Not that they are bad people. She didn't need them because she lived in a harmonious environment. I believe at this stage of our journey in reconstruction that what has been destroyed. We need this dictate, the dictate from the jungle.

Chapter 2

Why Do People Get Sick?

Welcome to the *new perspective of healing.*

"New," I said. But in reality, it is as old as Creation.

Yep, the subject is **healing.** You see it has to be as old as Creation. Because the components that are going to address healing or bring about healing has to be one that is considered native.

Geologically native plants are natural plants. **Natural plants are electrical.**

Why? The base of natural plants is the very foundation of what the Chinese called the C.H.O. arrangement. Carbon, hydrogen, and oxygen and I agree. So, for life to express itself into existence, there has to be what? **Carbon, hydrogen, oxygen.** What does the C.H.O. have to do with healing? It is the structure that would allow a substance to readily assemble biologically. Without carbon, hydrogen, and oxygen that substance is non-electrical. It is non-organic.

As we take a look at life. We want to clear the air. **We want to dismiss that myth.**

We want to expel the myth that "This and that is incurable." And that "This and that disease" came to the process of what? Germs? Virus or bacteria?

Well, you see this is a philosophy of medicine. As you can see, I am of a genetic predisposition that is African. **I am an African** and I'll take that! It is the greatest thing that ever happens to me to be born an African. Or if I was a China man, I would have loved to be a China man or a Caucasian or an Arab or an Eskimo. We are talking this way to show that whatever you are, that's what you were supposed to be. As we are that expression that carved out this image. I have no control over that!

So, as we travel on the journey of healing. We want to ask one question that hasn't been asked and I am totally unaware of it. It doesn't mean that it wasn't asked. **Why do we get sick?**

The body was not designed to be sick. Birds don't get sick. Elephants don't get sick. They need no vet. The lion doesn't need a vet. Neither does a giraffe or any of the natural animals. **WHY DO WE GET SICK?**

There has been a violation. A violation that is costing us our lives today. It would have been OK if I lived happily until I died. Because of the violations, that's not what's happening. Because of the violations, I became stressed. I became extremely stressed until I died. WHY DO WE GET SICK?! WHAT IS THE VIOLATION?! The violation comes with Creation, the understanding of it. The violation is when we have forgotten or dismissed Ecclesiastes when it is said "THE HERBS ARE FOR THE HEALING OF THE NATIONS." But we don't care about that GOD that made the statement that the herbs are good. We are conditioned for a chemical GOD.

So GOD, whatever you have to say is in trouble today.

Because I, pastor Gail (I'm referring to my brother), I've been a preacher for 30 years. GOD and my brother Fred "The Healer" came and showed me in the Bible, in the book of Genesis, Ezekiel, and Revelation that the herbs are for the healing of the nations. But what my brother Fred didn't know about me is that the food that I have been trained to eat has turned me against the very GOD that I claim to worship. I am compelled to violate the greatest image, the greatest structure. **GOD and the organic world.**

So now I don't want to take you into a crazy maze of a bunch of words that I am deploying to you. I want to make sense because you make sense. We all make sense. Why are we sick? And where is the violation?

Oh, I want to say this before I get into this subject. The reason for the violations, and they didn't come to me until I was about 50 years of age. I was born here in Ilanga, Honduras in a little village with seven houses. That little boy who is going to grow up in that village until the age of 8.

You mean to tell me from that position, in which the house I was born, was ground. It was the dirt. We didn't have ceramic or wood. Mama didn't have that. Mama had a dirt floor and it was always clean. So, from that level of being born in Ilanga, Honduras. To have made this leap into the understanding of things. I would arrive and deploy these words to you about health. The boy never went to school. The boy didn't read any books. I was the least candidate that could think about occupying a position that could be creditable. Well, guess what? Nature designs, and decides that violation, and you're going to see it.

I said we're going to travel on this journey. **It's a beautiful journey. It's a beautiful path.** It's peaceful because it brings understanding. Look carefully at the way that Africans lived in the jungle. Look at the way the Inca lived in the desert of Nasca. Look at the way the Maya lived in Central America. Then we go to the tropics and the Cultic in Mexico. Then we go to the Shoshone and the Skokomish, those are American Indians.

Carefully we're going to begin with the Africans, the Incas from South America, the Mayas central America, the Cultic from Mexico, and the American brothers and sisters' native. Do you know what we are called by a certain level of understanding? We're called the organic family.

All families are organic? NOT SO. I was in Nazca, Peru. I love Peru. I've been going to Peru since 1955. It was in Peru that I became aware of the organic family tree of Peruvian/Inca descendants.

He said "Blackman, are you aware of or do you have any idea what you represent?"

I said "No Pao."

He said "Well, we have something in common. We are a member of the organic family."

It's exactly what he said, it is organic. No waste, we do not produce waste. Everything about us is recyclable and this is why we didn't have any toilets.

Oh god, what is this? This man is showing me something that I never knew before. We didn't have any toilets. We didn't need that! Remember, what we ate were products that were considered native. No blood, uric acid, carbonic acid, or starch. You see when we ate, **we only ate electric foods.** That's all we had in our environment. The organic family only had electric food as part of their diet. They ate very little and were infrequent. It wasn't necessary to eat three times a day with a plate full of tajine, danshen, cassava, and blood. Not to mention the rice, which is starch, glycinate acid. No, we didn't have that. The organic family only ate electric foods. So, when he passes his feces, he can pass his feces in his hand and put it back in the soil.

But the family he said that lives outside of that cosmic arrangement. You don't want to be around when he uses the bathroom. It's something horrible. Imagine what goes on inside. It's what you smell. It's so unpleasant what goes on inside.

So, the organic family being that it was electric food is their diet. There was no waste. This was recyclable and didn't need a toilet. Do you understand Blackman what I'm saying to you? Of course, and I love it. The organic family was never diseased. Why? It was impossible because we live within the arrangement, the procession of life. I'm not an Inca, but certain things are indigenous to the Inca. I am not Maya, but I am an African and there is a connection with the family.

So, I was compelled to direct my thought pattern, my vision towards the continent. I am an African and what does that mean? It means that when Creation designed the African, there was food that was designed for that African. If you believe that this is untrue. Then let me take the diet of an African and give it to the man that lived on the ice, the Inuit. No! He was designed to eat whales and fish. **We were designed to eat something green** and nothing less. It is compatible with our genetic predisposition.

So now we come to "Why do we get sick?" The Africans had their food. The Eskimos had food. The Incas had food that you do not find in Africa. Nor what you find in Africa you won't find in Peru. What he needed was in Peru and what I needed was in Africa. If I ever make the mistake and select a component or a thought from another gene predisposition or another geography.

I'm only saying "Hey fellas, I am blind. I need to go to Kathmandu. I need to go to Nepal. I need to go to India or I need to go to Europe."

And what are you going there for?

You see I'm blind. I'm totally lost and being that I am lost. I don't know what is what and where to go. You see! We are blind and we show it.

I have friends that have books written by scholars from all over the world, from all religious structures. Scholars? I'm too ignorant about that. You see I was spared. I didn't go to school. So, the work of a scholar has no place in my environment. Why? Because what scholars do you know that have written a book to a people that addresses gene food consistency? Nobody! If we're going to violate the cosmic arrangement. All else is useless. It doesn't matter, you're violating! You are stressed.

What do you mean? There is such a thing as African food. And it isn't rice, beans, carrot, cow, chicken, hog, lamb, or goat. We didn't have that! Those things were brought to us. Those are the things that make us sick. The violations were done over the years. The African has been misled. Who do we, African people, point our fingers to? To say you are responsible. We don't know. But we know this! That we have been violated from a cellular structure and that is causing pain and anxiety among us. Stress! Stress so much we blow our own brain out and often in others and different ways and levels.

I am manic. But I contain it with my suit and ties and my cup of coffee. Not to mention my watch and my Mercedes. But one day very soon the doctor will say "Ay man, you got something on you, about you, in you."

"What is it doc? It is cancer?

Well, my ancestors didn't have cancer, it was unknown. Why do I have cancer? Well, **it's a virus.** The other one has AIDS, that's a virus. The other one, herpes, which is a virus. Everything happens to be a virus, germs, or bacteria. How do we know that? We don't know! Out of all the writers in the black community that we asked for. None of them paid attention to what we should have been paying attention to, **"Our health."** Our health, that would help me to love you and each other and myself.

First, our health was omitted. But we know all about the religious people. We know all about the cross. Jesus, we know all about that. But when we go home and eat. We eat something that would definitely offend our biological and cellular structure. Why is that? Where did that message come from? That we were supposed to eat starch and blood as our diet. When these things offend the Blackman's biology.

So today we are carving out a little path into the past. What we found is we are a member of the organic family. We didn't have any waste to rid ourselves of. But once in a while in New York or Los Angeles or anywhere you go. You'll see these trucks. Written on them, "Waste Management." How do you manage waste? I don't know. Afterall, it is waste. Why even manage it? Why produce it? This is the reason why we are sick.

So today we want you to know that we are a member of the organic family. Because of that level of understanding. We can put forth the effort to ameliorate much of the errors that beset us.

Isn't that beautiful? To come to that level of understanding that we need to change our diet. To which is compatible with our cellular predisposition, which is African. I'm not saying the African is better than the Caucasian or the African is better than the Chinese. When you start to compare races and groups then something has to be wrong with you. We are different. I am not a Caucasian. I am not a China man. I am an African. This means that I am compelled to follow that cosmic dictate and nothing should interfere with it. Do we now have the right to address this health situation that we are faced with Ebola?

Ebola? Cut it out. That's a joke. Africans have been dying for the last 500 years. The immunological system of an African has been compromised. Look at the diet of an African. None of it is African not to mention us. What do we do? Well, we fix it... That was the conversation that I had with my Mother before she passed.

She said "You know when you were a little boy, they used to ask me. What's Fred going to do?" I used to tell them "I don't know."

They asked my grandmother "Mama Hay, what's going to happen to Fred? What's he going to do?"

Mama Hay would say "I don't know." Well, why don't you send him to school?

That's when my grandfather would step in and said "Gorillas don't take their cubs to be trained by polar bears. He will not go to school! He has to learn what is consistent with his cosmic journey."

So, I went to the Motherland and selected these plants. And Wala! AIDS has been cured. Ebola has been cured. Diabetes, sickle cell anemia has been cured.

Why? Well, you know every plant lives by the dictate of their DNA that represents that plant. For instance, if I go to Burdock, I'm looking for iron. But if I go to the Lily Of the Valley, I'm looking for calcium and iron combined. If I want calcium in its purest form, I go to Sea Moss. If I want phosphorus, I go to the Sentaneto plant and so it goes with plants.

And so, it goes with animals and man. The food that we eat must be made by GOD. The cure has to be organic. Phosphate, carbonate, iodine, and bromide would ensure equilibrium in the body. It will begin to cleanse and revitalize. Stress would be demolished and a new direction will be presented to you.

So, I'm the little boy that didn't go to school and didn't understand why. But now I'm at that age, the winter stage. They wanted me to stay clean and that I would be able to absorb just the material that life has to offer. Not the philosophy of life. This is where we're going to end this chapter. That the Black man is not philosophical that comes from another society.

Philosophy has not done anything in ameliorating the condition of health or medicine. Is the existence of disease because of viruses, germs, and bacteria? So, we have to treat it with chemicals? Cyanide, oxide, mercury? That makes a lot of sense for philosophy. Which it isn't ours. We don't need philosophy. We are not philosophical folks. We are organic folks. The people that live by the philosophy produce waste.

Now we go to the organic family. What is the taught structure? There is none. I'm obedient and that's all. I have to be obedient to the laws of life. The arrangement of life. The elephant or giraffe doesn't live by a philosophy. He just obeys what mommy and pappi ate through generations of existence. So, it comes in now **"Honor thy mother and thy father that thy days may be long upon the land"** and that's what I did.

Chapter 3

Natural, Unnatural and the Supernatural

We're going to start with 3 categories: Natural, unnatural, and the third category I will not mention yet. Natural and unnatural. Why would we entertain unnatural things? Why would there be a category of unnatural? We're natural people. So, under natural, we're going to put Burdock in. Why? It is electrical! Do you know the Burdock plant? It grows in Chicago. It grows like mad all over the place. **It has energy, iron! It's electrical!**

Under the unnatural let's put Aloe Vera. What is the difference? You see the natural plants are made by GOD or nature. The unnatural plant is made by man. Therefore, there has to be a difference. The difference is when you select from an unnatural category or the unnatural state. You are introducing acid into somebody's body. You're not being truthful. Either because we're unaware or we were not helped by those that are supposed to help us.

Taught by students. So, he would give you Peppermint, Aloe Vera, Comfrey and they give you that! You go right now to Washington DC or Chicago some brothers and sisters are selling herbs. Who would sell you Peppermint? That's not natural. It would freeze the brain.

It's like giving someone sugar. When you give someone sugar, you don't like that person. You're showing them "I don't love you. I'm going to give you sugar." Why? It has **glycidic acid which will stimulate the body** and **cause you to be nervous.** But many of our brothers and sisters are still at that, as a medium to heal. Sugar?! In many forms. As a stabler is one of the ways that would be given to you.

Sugar cane, I used to love sugar cane juice. But it is deadly. It is not something that should go into our mouths. So, under the category of unnatural, we have those things. Let's add the hog that we eat. Why do we eat hog? Oh, because GOD made the hog. GOD did not make those things. Everything that GOD made was good. GOD did not make a mule. GOD did not make a horse. GOD did not make rice or beans.

They tell you about their history. Do you recall Menta the Jethro priest in England makes all of your beans? Just put that up there in the unnatural section.

Beans? Why not beans? There's starch there. All of the unnatural has starch. That's the one thing that they have in common. Anything that man-made must have starch. Starch is the binder. Starch is carbonic acid. Yet we eat it as food.

So, if I tell you that I don't like my neighbor. Something is wrong with me. Like I was when I married my third wife. I wanted to kill her and I wasn't joking. But apparently, I wanted to kill myself in 1963. That nigga was crazy and I ended up in the insane asylum in New Jersey in 1961. Why was I at an insane asylum with schizophrenia and paranoia? Because I was consuming all of the unnatural stuff. I didn't have anyone to really help me. Because everybody was telling me you need your beans, for what? Protein.

Protein? Now, what is that? We don't know. But we use the word "protein." Akeela Strough had sickle cell anemia. I deprived her of protein and I gave her iron. Now she no longer has sickle cell anemia. Why? Because there was a mineral that was missing in her diet and it's missing in all of our diets today. They call it "iron".

So, the other doctors noticed that I didn't give Akeela any hog, milk, meat, cheese, or eggs. She's jumping sky high.

"You have omitted protein from Akeela's diet?"

I said, "But Dr. Steinburg, I don't know what protein is."

"You don't know? And you are a so-called healer?"

"Well, I treat people with these herbs and they are healed after."

"You don't know what protein is?"

"I don't know."

"You're telling me, you are saying protein is unnecessary food?"

"I didn't say anything like that, I don't know what protein is."

"Well, it's one of the 19 amino acids, the building blocks of life."

"Amino acid? Protein is one of 19 amino acids the building blocks of life? No wonder! What does the body have to do with amino acids? The body lives in an alkaline environment."

Alkaline? The body doesn't need any acids. The acid eats you up. **Alkalinity preserves you.** It's electrical. Alkaline has life. I asked Dr. Steinburg "Is protein electrical?"

"I don't know."

I said, "You don't know?"

But you use that protein as your premise, as your foundation. I'm the uneducated and you're the educated. I've never been to school. So, I expect from you a different behavior. Is it electrical yes or no?"

"Well, I don't know."

"Well, that's good. Because there's a lot of things that I don't know and I will never know."

This prompts me to ask another question. "What is sickle cell anemia?"

"Well, sickle cell anemia is a disease that Black people got 10,000 years ago. They said the blood went through mutation."

I said, "I'm a little confused."

I'm more confused now than before! The reason is that there is a brother of ours with the name of Dick Gregory that goes around the world telling folks that GOD gave us sickle cells to fight malaria and you tell me it's a mutation.

But Dr. Steinburg, I want you to know this today. That sickle cell is neither GOD or mutation that Dick Gregory and you were saying. It is the deprivation of iron fluorine, that is sickle cell. I should know because the little girl no longer has sickle cell anemia. But they don't want to hear that, it's coming from a Blackman. An uneducated Blackman at that! I'm proud to say that, why? I am not a property of anyone's philosophy. I am a product of my Mama and my Grand Mama. I didn't have a father and that was good for me. Because I didn't have to fight between Mommy and Daddy to see which one is right.

All I had was Mama and came to find out. It was to be the very vehicle that I needed. The way that I was supposed to reach today, this goal in front of you. And I hope that I am the servant to you that my parents wanted me to be. So, make no mistake that today I am not in front of you condescending. Because I need you more than you need me.

So, understanding that life can only be found in an environment of Alkalinity. Why even have unnatural things? Why would that be necessary? Or wait, now we're going to take you to another song. They already took you from the natural to the unnatural. To get back from the unnatural to the natural, you just have to cross a thin line.

They create another category for you. The supernatural! Now how can there be a supernatural category? Just stick with the natural. No! They don't want the natural. They

want to take you to the unnatural and give you some carrot juice, beans, and pineapple. Nope, they're not through with us. So, they take us to the supernatural. You're not going to get away. What do you mean? You gotta be eating your chitterlings. Can you imagine this? Wait for a moment here.

Whenever an institution asks the people to eat food that they know is hurting you, is that love? Is that love?! That I know to be the truth.

Why would they do that? Look, I was down in Mexico. I saw an herb and I asked an herbalist.

"What herb is that?"

He said, "That's Damiana."

I said, "Can I have a kilo?"

He said, "No, I'm not going to sell you that herb."

I say "Why?"

He said "The license plate of your car."

I said, "What does the license plate of my car have to do with herbs?"

He said "Everything, your license plate said California and the best Damiana come from California. If I sell you mine, I'm not being truthful."

Look at the level of integrity of that Mexican.

Well, I'm driving down 3rd street in Memphis and I saw a line of folks trying to get into the store. Now, what are they selling in there? I don't know. But I stopped my car. When I got in there, I saw hog moss, chitterlings, pig snout, pig ears, selling that to us! They're telling you that "I don't like you, eat this!"

Come on now, I thought you love me. You know when I go in front of a Guru. He's not being truthful. Because when GOD put Black folks in Africa. Everything that Black folks needed was right there. GOD didn't put me in Africa and then he omitted a component that I need to go to Japan to eat or India, Europe, or Arabia. I don't need any of that and because I felt that I needed them.

"Lead me, please lead me, I need a leader. Can you see I need a leader! I'm blind, I need you to lead me."

But the leader instead of being truthful and kind and understanding. He tells me to eat beans, hog, and lamb. You don't love me or something is wrong with you. Look at the position, look at the abuse! I stood by for years and listened to that and watched that even today.

Nothing I can do. You think I feel good when I see a brother eat a lamb chop. You think I don't know the damage it's doing? I thought when I stopped eating the hog that I stopped eating that kind of worm that was very bad for me. So, I stopped eating the pork and I started eating the lamb and by eating the lamb it was 100x worse than pork. It has the Amtrac germs. You see they catch you going and they catch you coming.

So, in this category the super-natural. Some products go under the supernatural category to show you how imposing they are and inconsiderate. Look what they are going to do. The products under the natural can be seen.

The product under the unnatural, you can also see. But the product under the supernatural, mind, spirit, and soul you cannot see.

A little girl by the name of Makeena. See, we're going to talk about the truth now. Yes, we're going to share this today, truth! Makeena is sitting in the back of an automobile while her father is driving me to do a lecture in Los Angeles and another lecture was going to be in New York.

Makeena heard her brother ask me "What are you going to talk about today?"

I said, "I don't know."

"Well, when will you know?"

"When I get in front of the audience."

He said "Why don't you do me a favor. Why don't you talk about the Soul, Mind, and Spirit?"

The little 12-year-old girl said "You better not! You better not! Because you know I hate you. I hate you and I will always hate you."

And she had her reasons to hate me. Because I took away cheese, eggs, butter, and meat, the products that she likes so much. But the little girl had a vaginal discharge that wouldn't quit. And now she notices that even though she hated me for removing her ice cream, eggs, and milk her vaginal discharge stops.

She said "Even though I hate you. I like something about you. You tell the truth, but if you talk about the Soul, Mind, and Spirit, you are a liar."

A 12-year-old girl is going to talk to me like that? Yes, she did.

"You are a liar."

I said, "Why Makeena?"

"Because those things didn't come from reality, they came from imagination. They're unreal."

From that day onward, I'd stop. I thought that I was wrapped tight, but I wasn't. Because this 12-year-old girl was letting me know that I was saying things I thought or believed that I know.

As a healer, I cannot live in the zone of belief. I have TO KNOW or I DON'T KNOW! Because if I intended to give you Molend, but instead I give you Fox Straw because they look alike, I will kill you. Because I believed it was Molend, but it was Fox Straw.

You cannot work as a healer in that world. In an environment of belief. You got to know or you don't know. So Makeena stopped me from being a liar. And I used to use it. I'm spiritual and I'll go home and eat some glazed ham. But I'm spiritual! What makes me so different from those who aren't? I claim I'm spiritual. You see, it doesn't make me better than you. That doesn't happen. So, see all of these kinds of stuff over here in the unnatural and supernatural have to be omitted.

I decide to go on a journey with that Black woman in the jungle of Africa and I begin compounding these plants using only Alkaline plants. Why? Because I want to make sure. I don't want to cheat you. I don't want to lie to you.

I don't want to come in front of your face or your brothers with something other than the truth. And the truth is what you know, not what you believe.

So, the boy got a job as a steam engineer making all kinds of money and he's going to quit his job. The uneducated boy that didn't go to school should be happy to have an engineering job.

No! That Mexican put me on a journey that I could not stop. Because he said, "Stop eating for 94 days."

I stopped eating and when I went back and saw that Mexican. That Mexican said to me "This is you."

"What do you mean?"

"Anyone that fasts for 90 days never go back to the old life again. You're going to be a slave to the plants."

I was 30 years of age. My steam engineer job had turbines and gages of all kinds. I can read them. Oh boy, I don't like this anymore. I decided to buy a book on biochemistry and pathology and biology. I began to study these books. 10 years I worked for the county, 10 years I studied that science. All 3 of them biochemistry, biology, pathology, and at the end of the 10th year. The first man that was cured was Mr. Federick he was blind for 11 years and he was seeing in 2 days. He brought his daughter with him. She had epilepsy. She was cured in the first treatment. When that happened. Oh, I was happy people were being cured. I quit my job. All my friends cried and me too. Cause I loved them. There were White engineers, Filipinos engineers, Japanese and Blacks. And we all were in love. I miss them.

I said, "I got to go."

The boss said, "Are you out of your mind?"

I said, "I may be."

"You've been 10 years on the job and you have 10 more to go and then you can retire."

I said, "I can't stay, I got to go."

Because I noticed the mistake that our healers were making. They were integrating herbs that were natural and unnatural. You don't mix them, you'll neutralize both. You do not mix acidity and alkalinity.

The boss said "You know I'm going to give you a letter that if you fail in your journey of healing. You can come back within five years with the same seniority."

That white man Brett Howard is a German. I said, "Thank you."

He said, "Because I see that you are deliberate."

I said "Well Brett Howard, it's either win, lose or draw. I don't care, I'm going."

7 years later, he was looking at the television and he saw me being arrested. Practicing medicine without a license. Selling products that weren't approved by the FDA and claiming to cure AIDS and other diseases. Which they accuse is a fraudulent claim. How did he know I was making a fraudulent claim? Was I going to leave my life in the country of Honduras to come to the United States to put lies in the newspapers? And my Mama is alive and my face is in front of the public and I'm representing Africa.

Because I am an African. I am not an Afro-American, I'm not a hybrid. I am an African born in America. Now with this African, I begin to do the research. I found out that we cannot eat the same food that the Caucasian or Indian eats. Indians can eat beans. They call it the calcify button that is very dangerous for us.

Arabs can eat lambs. That's fine, let them do that while they're drinking their coffee. We can't do that, it hurts us. We're not against anyone. All we're doing is showing that the difference that we are has not been treated. This is why we tend to be angry and to overlook certain things. Then we use these measurements that confuse things for instance.

You know Chicago, Elijah Mohammed, Nat King Cole. Which one is better? King? These are men that fit in the equation. So, you cannot compare one against the other. Each one came with a message. I'm different from all of them and I will continue to be different. I've cured AIDS! If that doesn't mean anything, it's only scratching the surface.

Mr. G. the cameraman came with his sister who had lupus and was dying. She's cured. Does that make me know everything in healing? So, the journey into the healing path. We begin to see that it is not about using a yardstick good and bad. Up and down. You cannot compare a lion with a tiger. They are different animals, totally different not to be compared with. So, I want you readers to know that I'm not here talking about things that you don't already know.

Chapter 4

The Conversation

Q.- Can you tell us a little bit about yourself? An introduction for the readers.

H.- I was born in a small village name Ilanga in Spanish Honduras in 1933. The boy grew up never going to school. Whether it's Kindergarten, Grade School, High School, or whatever. I became a merchant seaman. By the time he became a merchant seaman he was very deadly ill. He had asthma from birth. He was impotent at 28. At 30 he had diabetes, asthma, obesity, and insanity. With the help of the Mexican people. I was cured. I decided to enter the field of natural medicine.

Q.- Can I inject you for a quick second. When you start, you refer to yourself as a third person, then you switch yourself to the first person. Do you see who you were earlier in your life as a different person as though you became yourself in the second half of your life?

H.- I was always a different person. I disagree with EVERYTHING! Everything I heard I disagree with. I have been working since I was 11. Because my

Grandmother raised me and she was my responsibility. My duties were to take care of paying the rent, buying her clothes, and buying her food.

I was tall. I was supposed, "Sensible." So, I just grew up and at the age of 14, I made a statement. That I was going to do something to help humanity. But when I made that statement. I also knew that I was going to come up against the established or prevailing philosophy of life. That I knew at 14 years of age. But I didn't know that one day I would be that person known as the Healer.

Before I became a Healer. I didn't have a girlfriend until I was 21 years of age. I disagree with what I saw and even now with my interrelationship with women. I don't believe that there is a woman that could rightfully say that she loves me. Because of the way I've lived and the way I see things and I'm not really upset about it.

About that, I live differently. I see things differently. I feel different and I don't share that with most people. Because it's so far away. You know you don't want to disturb anyone. Even the healing I bring on to the world.

My very first patient...I was a steam engineer worker for the port of Los Angeles. This blind man has heard that I was experimenting with these plants and his neighbor said "Why don't you take it." He took the plant and in two days he was seeing. He was blind for 11 years and that shook me. Cause I couldn't explain to the world the mechanic behind this blind man seeing.

Q.- What were your thoughts when formulating the compound?

H.- The way that the compound came into existence. Being a steam engineer, I knew the PH value. The PH factor had a lot to do with healing. But the herbalist then, like the herbalists today, are unaware that the PH factor has a lot to do with it. Meaning this,

I said that "If GOD tells us that the herbs are for the healing of the nations in the book of Genesis, in the book of Ezekiel, in the book of Exodus and the book of Revelation. It said that the herbs are for the healing of the nations."

Then as I go further into the history of medicine. This is what I found that the great Hippocrates used herbs to cure diseases and he cured every disease known to man. This man was curing every disease in Greece, 365 years before Jesus Christ was even born. So, when people tell us only Jesus heals. You remind them that Hippocrates was healing long before he was born.

So I said, "If Jesus cured with herbs. Hippocrates cured with herbs. And GOD said, "The herbs are for the healing of the nations." What's up? Why aren't we curing with herbs today?"

So, one day before I went to work. My wife and I were talking all night. We were engaged in this conversation about these herbs. My wife said to me that there could be something locked in someplace that prevents us from accomplishing the goals that

Jesus Christ and Hippocrates accomplished. When I went to work that night, I found it.

At last! I was so happy. I was extremely happy. Because I said it is required of us to maintain the PH of 6.9 in the boiler at work. At 7 PH which is the neutral zone. We have to keep it slightly on the acid side which is 6.9 PH. The reason why we maintain the PH at 6.9 is to keep the tube of the boiler clean. At 6.9 PH there will be no life form. But if the PH is 7.1, oh! Now you're going to experience life. Life forms would begin to form in the tube of the boiler preventing the radiant heat or the convection heat from reaching the tube.

I said that "If life was so powerful that it could exist in the temperature of 450*. Then the herbs that heal will have to be alkaline on 7+ PH instead of acid 6.9 PH."

Then I begin to check all the PH levels of all the herbs.

I begin to test it. I tested Comfrey, acid. I tested garlic, acid. I also tested Aloe Vera, St. John Wort, Rose Hips, Comfrey all of these things are very acidic. Carrot juice is extremely acidic. Yet the healers in New York then and now still recommend these acidic foods.

So, I said, "Well, let me investigate further and see which are the alkaline herbs."

And I began to see that Burdock, Yellow Dock, also the Elderberry, these are alkaline plants. Also, the Virginia Snakeroot, that's alkaline.

One has to know the herbs that are alkaline, opposed to the herbs that are acid. This today is not really considered nor do they follow that particular road or understanding. Because the herbalist of today is reconnecting Peppermint. Peppermint is VERY acid! Peppermint freezes the brain. Some even recommend Peppermint Oil. Peppermint oil is extremely costly.

Now we have this kind of information in front of us being dissimulated and carried out. So, there's confusion in the population. But the one thing that my supporters of the people that helped me, that counsel me.

They said to me "The one thing that you have in your favor is that you have cured and you are curing diseases that others are not curing."

There is a barometer that tells us that the acid herbs used is preventing them from reaching the goals they're pursuing.

It was my steam engineering experience that helped me in biology to understand the herbs that GOD made. Yes! It has to be made by GOD. If we eat something that GOD didn't make, we are at risk of disease. Then we're going to be angry like I was at 30 years of age. I was extremely angry!

So, I didn't know that I would, but my mother wanted me to be a preacher and I didn't want to go to church.

I said, "Who me? Be a preacher? I don't want to be a preacher."

And look what I'm doing now. Look what I'm doing! I called my mother on my birthday two days ago. She was laughing.

She said, "You see what I wanted you to do? You're doing it! Only because people are being healed that is the work of a Shepherd."

Q.- As a young man, you had a sense that you can heal people. But you didn't know quite how you would do it. Then in your 20s, you started to look into herbs?

H.- No, I didn't look into herbs in my 20s. I didn't know anything about herbs in my 20s. I made a statement at 14 years of age that I was going to do something to help humanity. But I didn't know it was going to turn out to be these herbs. So, when I was sick at the age of 30 and I got help from a Mexican. Then I proceeded to pursue it.

I was working as a steam engineer at the time. Every day I would go to work and GOD would talk to me and said "How could you be healed of all those dreadful diseases and you're going to hold that from humanity?" And I would go to work and see these turbines, condensers, and these boilers and I would get so angry. And that's when I stepped up my research.

Q.- Why would you get so angry?

H.- Because I wanted to get away from them. Because I wanted to go into the herbs. But I was then 47 years of age and I was 10 years in the job. I had seniority. I was making a lot of money, and I had a wife with two babies with one on the way.

I quit my job! GOD said "You're going to quit! If you're going to starve, you're going to die starving. But you're going to quit this job."

I left and I was put in jail. You know the whole thing that happens to me in New York. I was arrested in St. Martin one night and I was taken to jail.

Oh, it's been a journey. It's been nice. Because it was like a test. I remember being down to only $400 when I started this business. I only have $400 and I started this healing journey with $400 and here I am today.

A little girl in New York named Hija was brought to us with a hole in her heart, she is now 16. And another little girl that was brought to me from Atlanta was blind from the age of 8 to the age of 11 with a tumor on her frontal lobe. She no longer has a tumor on the frontal lobe, her name is Meca. There's a little girl in Minnesota, her name Akeela Strough. She no longer has sickle cell anemia.

A month ago, I gave a lecture in New York and a young lady came forth and said "I don't have lupus anymore!"

So, this kind of thing tells us that we the Black race have the answer to the world's health. We have the answer to the disease state. But we are afraid to take that responsibility. Because we live in fear. We fear! We're scared of the White man. We're scared of GOD. We say that we fear GOD, I don't know why we fear GOD?

Q.- Is it possible for one group to have a cure for the world? Because part of your outlook or beliefs is that people are at their healthiest when they are eating food that comes from the region of their ethnic origin.

H.- That's not happening.

Q.- That's what you believed?

H.- I don't believe that either. What I believe is to eat foods that come out of the product of life itself. I don't care if you're Chinese, Eskimo, or Arab or what. If you eat something natural, you're going to be healed.

Q.- Do you believe that certain people, for instance, black people should not eat foods that are not natural to them?

H.- Oh, that's a horse of a different color. Black people should not eat Chinese food or even Caucasian food. There was a book out by a man known as Pablo Iiola. He is known to be one of the most distinguished nutritionists in the world. He said that if your ancestors are from Africa, your body is not programmed to digest milk. But if you're European, yes. So right there, they're telling us that there's a different genetic makeup of these two individuals.

Q.- So if people have different genetic makeup which makes them react differently to different herbs and food products. Would it be possible for one group to have a cure for the entire world or would they be more towards a cure for people within the same ethnic group?

H.- Well it should be like that, I suppose. Our experience shows us that it crosses all boundaries. Because all people come to us. I recall a time when more White people were coming to us. Chinese and Japanese also come to us. My wife cured a woman in Japan of lung cancer and she never seen the woman. They called from Japan and told my wife about their illness. She sent them compounds and she was cured. Annet has cured many, so did Tatanisha and they've never seen these people. We sent compounds to Europe and they were cured.

I have a letter from a psychiatric group in France who wants me to go and give a lecture to them. Why? Because someone with schizophrenia was cured that I didn't know about. So, these compounds cured everything whether you're Black, White, or Eskimo. Providing natural things, the substance that you're going to eat as a staple. Yes! As we would do, you are 100% right. It has to be genetically consistent with you.

Q.- I like to hear more about the relationship or our staple diet and where our ancestors are from?

H.- We're going to give you an example. A good example from the day that GOD created this universe and made Black people. How many years has it been since GOD placed Black people in Africa? Do you have any idea? The anthropologist has no idea. But they will sprout out these numbers for you, that GOD made the universe 9.5 billion years ago.

So, the other is: When did he put Black people in Africa? They say 1.5 million years ago. And what was the food that GOD placed in Africa for these people? Certainly, it could not have been the potato, rice, beans, yam, chicken, hog, or cow. It could not be goat or lamb. Because all these things are hybrid. GOD did not make these things. These things came just recently only 4000 years ago. So, what were they eating in Africa before we were taken away? What were we eating in Africa before the invasion of men from Europe? We simply don't know and it's because we are unaware of this diet that GOD made specifically for us. That's why we are so angry today and why we're so divided.

Everybody is laughing at us. They are laughing more at me. On the airplane, the pilot came to see me two weeks before 9/11. They were looking at a brochure I had that said AIDS has been cured. An herbalist cured AIDS and the Supreme Court of New York can't deny or disagree. They were laughing at me. Why? Because you are not supporting me. So, they think that I'm a fake.

Because if it was a White man curing AIDS.

The captain said, "The whole White race would be supporting them."

But my race is not going to support me. The leaders of America can't do it. Farrakhan can't do it. Jesse Jackson can't do it. Because they were not designed to do these types of work. They were designed to lobby and talk. And to the likes of Mr. Al Sharpton, he likes to make people march. That's cool. But we have a job to do in healing the Black race. Now, that comes in a different category. **Those leaders cannot help me and that's why I'm vulnerable.**

Q.- In what ways do the Black race need healing?

H.- One of the areas the Black race needs healing most is in the central nerve system. Because we have been eating acid food for 500 years.

Q.- How does that manifest itself in terms of socially or physically?

H.- Socially we see that very seldom that the leaders agree with themselves. The leaders are at war. They're all in disagreement. Because among the leaders you find Muslims, Christians, Buddhists, and all of that. And they all seem to disagree with each other's position.

Q.- How about the politician?

H.- The politician? Well, I don't know what role politics plays in our progression of health. How we see it again, is that we are not together on any pragmatic issues, that are going to elevate us in producing something for our own existence. Self-preservation is the first law of nature and we are the only people on the planet that denied that.

Q.- Can you elaborate a little more about the relationship between diet and behavior.

H.- Diet and behavior have a direct relationship.

Q.- Is this affecting Black Americans in a particular way? Is that something you can see throughout our community and would the difference be that Black Americans are not in their original homeland? Would that be why there would be a greater problem for Black Americans?

H.- Temperature and food. But not so much for an African. Do you know that Black America on a scale from 1-10, if we are to be perfect at ten, Black America is about five, Africa is about two. Black America is closer to the goal than Africa.

Q.- Are you saying diet or behavior?

H.- Diet and behavior. Because if a young man in California is in love with you. He's not going to ask you what tribe you are a member of, right? No, he's not.

Q.- Right.

H.- But in Africa, if you are a "Susu" and I'm a "Malaki." I'm not going to marry you because I'm supposed to be your enemy. But they're both Black! You see in America the brother is not going to ask you what tribe you're a member of. He's going to marry you because he likes you, right?

Q.- Is it better to have your offspring to be linked at least in traditional society or to certain Geological regions or not being removed from the area where the vegetation that was designed for them to eat, and you won't have the problem that you describe?

H.- Good! That would be good and I agree with you. But there's one other part of it. The African people are eating Cassava, and Cassava is cyanide. Pure cyanide unadulterated. You didn't have any of that and it's because you didn't have the cyanide you were able to produce plastic (George Washington Carver). You were able to build The White House, produce electricity, and produce agriculture. The African man and no other Black man in the world has ever done that. That shows that Black Americans, even though taken away from the motherland and given meat, which is responsible for our anger. We are still able to do things that are over and above any other race in the world.

The Black race has proven that and now that another one comes. Your brother and servant, me. It is not so surprising that he cured AIDS. Sickle cell is like play for me. Diabetes? We cure 10 a month. Are there any centers in the United States that cure diabetes? WE cure diabetes! What are they going to do now? I would like to hear the excuse. I would like for someone to take this particular entity to the leaders of America and I would like to hear the excuse they are going to give us for not supporting it.

Chapter 5

The Interview

Q.- If we want to lose weight in a fast and healthy manner how do we do that?

H.- Well to answer your question. I've been struggling with weight since 1964. I was 291 pounds and now I only weigh 120 and I'm 6"2. I wanted to know what it would be like on the other side of being big and I wanted to see the benefits of it. Because I've been told that there are such things as the standard weight per height measure. But we cannot live by those measures. I weigh 120 pounds and trust me. I've not felt this good my entire life.

Approximately eight months ago, I stopped eating for 64 days. But I made a mistake because I had a speech to do in Philadelphia. By not eating for those 64 days, I was going for 90 days. But I remember I had a speech to do in Philadelphia. So, when I went to do the speech, I fainted. I had to faint! Because I was talking too long and I was not eating for 64 days. What I've done was to discontinue anything that had glucose. **Glucose is the underlying enemy.**

Whenever you indulge in it, it would be difficult to lose fat.

I lived in Honduras and California. In Honduras, I discovered a plant known as Corsica. Corsica is a plant that the Maya used and they used another one known as "Tail-wa-sin-tay". I eat those plants. Those plants do not have starch or glucose. You're going to look at your body losing weight and you're going to be frightened.

Q.- What did you do during the 64 days that you didn't eat to sustain the energy level to operate?

H.- Well I was in the village of Usha in Honduras. We have thermal water with a PH level of 9.8. This means that this substance has a high level of oxygen and it's the oxygen that the body needs. Not rice, beans, or a piece of meat. It needs oxygen. That is the fuel of the body. So, I drank the water and I would eat the Corsica. This is a plant that I just discovered that the Mayas used to eat. It is delicious, it tastes like cucumber. So, I ate the Corsica plant and drank the water and that was it.

Q.- Did you have a routine while you were fasting and traveling?

H.- I have a lot of work to do. Directing programs, building huts, the electric culture program. So, I was busy. You'll be surprised what water does. I learned to use the waters in Ecuador. For the people of Vilcabamba, their diet is 78% water and 22% solid. Because the body doesn't need that solid food. It needs fuel and the fuel comes from oxygen and water.

Q.- How do you compare the water in your village of 9.8 PH to the water we have here in the United State?

H.- **Well 9.8 is a very high level of PH, It's Hydrogen ion concentration. A high level of PH ensures that you have the amount of oxygen that the body needs. After finding the minerals in the thermal waters you discover the benefit of bathing in it. In America, there is Trinity water. Trinity water is thermal and it is 9.8 PH.**

Q.- So you're 82 years old and you're still making babies, can you explain that?

H.- **Change the diet!** **All men can do it! What I did was to depart from the usual diet that mostly men indulge in. Remember I was impotent at 30. How was it that I was impotent at 30 and I'm making babies in my 80s? See what happens? It's the information! I got it in 1964 and many brothers and sisters may not have received that message yet. That message came from a Mexican. The Mexican was showing gene food consistency. Meaning your cellular predisposition determines what you should eat.**

When I went to Mexico, I had already traveled to Russia, Saint Petersburg, London, Spain, and many places in Africa.

I was asthmatic. I was impotent. I had diabetes. I was in fact CRAZY. I was placed in an insane asylum in 1961 with schizophrenia and paranoia.

So, I went to Mexico and the man asked me "Where are you from?"

I said, "I'm from Honduras."

He said, "We cannot talk."

I said, "Why?"

"Because Black folks don't come from Honduras. Maya comes from Honduras. So, where are you from?"

"Oh, I'm from Africa."

Now we're talking. Now because you are from Africa. Do you believe GOD was drunk when he put Black people in Africa?

I said "No."

"Well do you believe he put a diet there for you?"

I said "Sure."

And what's the diet? Rice, beans, potatoes, yam, cow, hog, and lamb.

He said "Not so! That's not a diet of an African. What is the diet of an African? All that which is native."

But I didn't know there's such a thing. Because I was a Muslim, you know I was Islam. Islam gave me a whole lot of good things. I met Elijah Mohammed. I met the messenger talking to him like I'm talking to you. But the messenger's information at the time needed a little bit more help. So, he told me that I could not eat meat any longer. No lamb, I could not drink milk and abstain from all these things and here I am now at 82. I'm as happy as I've ever been in my life.

Q.- Can you tell me about the relationship and the work you did with Michael Jackson?

H.- I was home on a Sunday afternoon in Los Angeles. Someone threw a rock at my window. When I looked and it was Randy. I've known Randy over the years. Randy Jackson, Michael Jackson's brother. So, he came upstairs.

"What's up?"

"My brother wants to see you."

I said "Who?"

"Michael"

"Michael wants to see me?"

I'm the least of an individual that people want to see. I'm at the bottom of the totem pole. I went to see him and he agreed to me traveling with him. I told him that I would be able to help him. He couldn't sleep. He was in a bad, very emotional state.

Q.- What time frame was this?

H.- 2004, I was with him from February until September. At the end of September,

I told him, "You know you're singing. You feel good, you're looking good. I'm leaving."

He said, "Don't leave me."

I said, "Why?"

He said, "I want you by my side."

But I have a business to build. I love Michael, Michael was a beautiful brother.

Q.- What did you do for him?

H.- What I did for him was this: I gave Michael intracellular chelation, which means that I'm going to clean every cell that makes up any organ that totals his biological structure. Because he was on a whole lot of drugs, you know pharmaceutical drugs. He couldn't sleep because his nerve was shattered. So, I began treating him. At the end of the period, he was doing good and I left.

Q.- How did you learn how to do these things? In 1987 you were charged in New York City with practicing medicine without a license. You were ultimately charged, indicted, and taken before the New York Supreme Court and you won that case. The charge was practicing medicine without a license and claiming that you cured AIDS, cancer, diabetes. So, the question is: How did you win that case? Against what some people say it's the toughest prosecutors in the land?

H.- Well, it was 1987 the 10th of February. My mother knew they were coming when I told my mama that I've cured my 13th AIDS patient. She said, "They are going to get you!"

Q.- Let me stop you there. You said, "I've cured my 13th AIDS patient." So, you had 13 patients that had AIDS and you say, you "cured them"?

H.- So my mother said, "They are going to get you."

But I said, "Mom, why are they going to get me?"

"Because you must remember that you live in a society that supports a certain philosophy and a certain system. You being the color you are, Black, and then you're going against the grain. They're going to get you!"

So, I'm in my office on February the 10th, and here comes the detective. You're charged with practicing medicine without a license. Selling products that are not approved by the FDA and claiming you cured AIDS and other diseases. I said "Yes." Well, you are making a fraudulent claim. I said to the detective "How do you know that?"

Q.- Because you were advertising in the newspapers?

H.- Of course I was advertising in the Village Voice, Amsterdam News, and the New York Post.

Q.- And you were telling people that you cure AIDS, sickle cell, lupus, herpes, blindness, diabetes, paralysis, and others.

H.- So they knocked on my door and took me to jail. But the funny thing about it, I was happy! I was very extremely happy when everybody in my office was crying. I was happy because my Mama told me they were coming and I know I had sufficient evidence to prove my position. Not only scientific. Imperatively, historically and which every way they desire.

So, when I was in jail. I'm saying what defense would they have against me? I would like to know. But I didn't blame the attorney general, Mr. Robert Abrams. Because why should he expect from me the statement that I cured AIDS, sickle cell, and blindness. When no one else has ever made those claims. The man had a right to arrest me. But he was making a mistake. So, I'm sitting in jail and I'm happy. I went in front of a Judge. I asked 3 questions.

Q.- You defended yourself!?

H.- Of course I did!

Your honor!

"Is it a fact that the Holy Bible teaches that the herbs are for the healing of the nations?" She said yes.

"Is it a fact that science shows that the human body is carbon-based?" And to complement a carbon-based substance, you need a natural substance.

Because the body only accepts the substance through the process known as chemical affinity. Chemical affinity is important, it's an electrical transfer. The body can only accept what it's made of, not something new or alien to it.

"Your Honor! Is it a fact that the father of medicine Mr. Hippocrates, the man that established the principles of medical science today, cured every disease known to man...Did he use herbs or chemicals?" She said herbs.

I said, "Thank you very much, I rest my case."

So, I understand that the state was unprepared to defend itself. They were unprepared because in the past there were 2781 cases that came before the

Supreme Court and lost. I won. Not only did I prove scientifically. But I had the diagnostic sheets and I do have them today and those diagnostic sheets didn't come from me. They came from their school. Their medical accredited school.

Q.- Were there some requirements for you to actually bring patients into court from each of those maladies? And you brought multiple patients into court, who want to testify themselves. You also had medical records showing that they were a victim of the disease and then showing that it had been cured by one doctor and a second doctor verifying what the first doctor had said.

H.- Yes! We have to remember this: that whenever you make a statement that goes against the grain. You better be prepared! The Judge said that I have to bring one of every patient that I cured and there was one that said "other." The other was a man that came from Italy. He was paralyzed. I was supposed to take nine, I took 77. I know that my brain was not the same as your brain or any other brain. We're unique. So, when I make a statement. They are going to take my statement and put it against philosophy. It doesn't fit. I represent an entity that is not philosophical.

Q.- That entity is?

H.- Well, it's an African one. I'm an African and we have to remember that! You see, we think that we can take a philosophy of the European or Chinese and intricate that into an African brain. That does not resonate! It cannot resonate! You cannot be yourself when you've been adulterated. Being that I am an African. I'm going to look at things the African way. The African way seems to reduce things to the least common denominator and guess what I found? That there is only one disease, not two, not three, ONE!

When I opened my big black mouth and told the Judge that. Oh my god, what did you say?

I said, "Your Honor there's only one disease."

Could you substantiate that? Of course, I'm not just going to deploy a bunch of empty words. I represent a country. I represent people. I represent a race and I represent myself. I'm not going to undermine myself. There's only one disease.

The Judge said, "What is it?"

I said, "You already know."

She said, "Try me."

It was a woman, Ann Thelmon.

I said, "Your Honor when someone has sinusitis what is obstructing the nasal passage?

She said, "Mucus."

And another has bronchitis, what is obstructing the bronchial tube?

She said, "Mucus"

And when another has pneumonia what's covering the cells of the lung?

She said, "Mucus."

Dr. Victor Herbert who is defending the state of New York jumped up and said, "What about AIDS?! You and your one disease theory."

I said, "Your Honor, this doctor said I believe in a theory. I am the last individual on earth that could believe in a theory. I do not lend myself to theories or philosophy. Either I know or I don't know."

He's talking about theories. I'm talking about reality, not theories, not philosophy.

So, she said, "What about AIDS?"

She wants to know, where's the mucus?

I said "Your Honor have you been to an AIDS ward?

She said, "Yes."

What is it that an AIDS patient spits up every five minutes? Mucus!

Where is the mucus? It's in the skin. It's in the blood and in the lymphatic system that makes up the immune illogical system. That is where you find the mucus, Mr. Victor Herbert. How can you disagree with the truth?

You see what happened is I didn't go to school. I have never been to school. I have never attended school. Kindergarten, grade school, high school, or anything. But I had parents that kept me anchored to the African way. Not to the Chinese way. Not to the European way. Not the Japanese way. I am an African.

Q.- Were your patients all of color?

H.- No, I have patients that are White. I have more White patients than I have Blacks.

Q.- AIDS, can you walk us through the step-by-step process. Where you have a patient that has AIDS and you do XYZ and then the patient no longer has AIDS. Can you guide us through that?

H.- Of course, the first patient was a brother in Boston named Michael White. His sister was from DC.

She said "My brother-in-law has AIDS and he's from Boston. So, what can you do?"

Well, I'm going to send him the compound. The compound that I made was made to cleanse the cells. It comes in the category of phosphate, carbonate, iodide, bromide. Now we're entering the science of biochemistry. These are foods and vitalizes. I removed from the man's diet: Lactose, uric acid, carbonic acid, milk, starches, and meat. By removing these things from his diet and then cleansing his cells. He begins to see recovery in 24hrs and so it went. They kicked him out of the hospital in Boston. Then there was a young woman in DC. Thelma Peterson was her name. She was the one that introduced me to my second AIDS patient. From then it was all the way, all the way alive.

Q.- Now you have documents?

H.- I have proof now. I have folders with the documents in them, diagnostic sheets.

Q.- And the medical world still puts out that you are a quack, a crazy man, you're not credential, and that you run scams on people. But you have documented proof that you heal people. So, when you get patients, do the patients need to come to see you in person?

H.- **No, in fact, we send out a thousand packages a day throughout the world to Israel, Hong Kong, China, Russia. We send packages all over the world. You don't have to go to Honduras. But because the thermal waters are there and they accelerate your healing when bathing in it and drinking it.**

About medical science saying that I'm a quack. I do not blame medical science for making that statement. Because my race had never done anything on that level of endeavor to express itself. Able to cure diseases on that level in other words. So sure, I'm a quack. But I don't care what they say. What I am concerned with is not medical science. Because I know that they are the ones that are violating. I am not the violator. Hippocrates did not establish the school of medicine by using chemicals. Chemicals cannot assimilate with the human body, but herbs can. Because herbs are electrical and we have yet to understand that.

I was concerned with the Black leadership of America, not medical science. When I have cured these people of sickle cells, lupus, herpes, and blindness, I was happy. Now I can go to all the leaders. Not so! They are not interested in the healing of any Black people.

Q.- That's an explosive claim.

H.- That is not an explosive statement! That is the reality. There isn't a Black leader in America that is interested in the health of the Black race.

Q.- You say that because they refuse to interact with you?

H.- They are not in the position to respond! If they were, my first case of AIDS was cured in 1984. Since then, we have been curing people of lupus, cancer, herpes, and blindness. Not one Black leader came over and said "Let us help a brother out." Hahaha!

Q.- You just mention the C word, cancer. I know people that are going through chemotherapy and they talked about how devastating those treatments were. So, you obviously do not treat with chemo. Why is it wrong or is it wrong for a cancer patient to be treated with chemotherapy?

H.- Chemotherapy is an approach that destroys cells. Chemotherapy does not distinguish the good cells and bad cells. It just destroys cells. It's an acid approach. My approach is Intra Cellular cleansing. What causes disease in the first place? An acid condition. Well then let's sweep it out. Let us find the plants that are consistent with cleansing. You see we just begin to wake up. We just begin to realize that we are in a deep deficit.

Q.- What do you mean by that?

H.- Well, I mean we have never spent time analyzing or even trying to understand the difference

in our genetic predisposition. We have never understood the science of biochemistry. All of the folks that had come to us, they come to us with histories. Bunch of histories, lots of religions, a lot of philosophy. But none of them came with food that would help me to live as healthy as I possibly can.

Look carefully, we're not going to make excuses anymore. Because if we continue to make excuses. We're going to go deeper into the deficit. Just recently a report came out that the Christian diet needs to be examined. Because in the Christian's diet there are people eating hog, potatoes, rice, and beans. But if we take these substances to a biochemist, he's not going to find any food in these substances. So why do we eat these things? Then we get sick. I always use that Black woman in the jungle for some reason, she keeps showing up. This Black woman in the jungle keeps showing up and setting a standard and raising the bar. Why?

Q.- Tell me what you refer to when you say this "Black woman in the jungle?"

H.- I mean this sets a standard. This woman didn't die because of the disease. She didn't have any hospitals in the jungle. She didn't have any doctors or medicine. That's why Hippocrates said that "Your food should be your medicine." Because the African people didn't have doctors. They didn't have any of the substances that would violate the biology of the individual. So how long did they live? Do you and I know how long those Africans lived in the forest of Africa before the chemical people came? Furthermore, my Mama wasn't naked, she was natural. To say my mama was "naked" in the forest of Africa is to say GOD made clothes.

Q.- I remember an interesting interview CBS did on Lisa "Left-Eye" Lopez. Can you please tell us what your experience was with her? Because we have the footage that she was committing to spreading the word about you. What did you do with her and for her?

H.- I don't know why Lisa said she would spread the word about me. Because she healed me.

Q.- She healed you?

H.- That's right! This young lady came to me because she needed help. Her eyes were blinking really fast and she had a little thing that she was suffering from that she wanted to get rid of, and she got rid of them. One day she said something to me. It was 4 a.m. She was on a 21 day fast, no sorry 42-day fast. Lisa came into the hut where I was living with these 2 cups of sea moss. Sea moss is known as Chondrus Crispus. I had her drinking sea moss. She said, "You know you have helped me, but you need healing." And she was right! I was in a state of disarray and I didn't know it. It took a woman to show me that and Lisa was the one that showed me.

Q.- What do you mean you were in a state of disarray?

H.- At the time. I was involved with three different wives. I had three wives then. My life was not stable because I got another woman pregnant. A young girl 19 years old was pregnant outside of those three wives. So, Lisa said to me that I need help and I didn't know how much help I needed until Lisa told me that morning, and she was right.

Q.- What was the kind of help you needed?

H.- I was emotionally out of it.

Q.- Did you realize that you were finding temporary security, affection, or love through the act of these other women?

H.- Love? No, love is something that I never depended on from a woman. In fact, I don't even like it. listen carefully.

Q.- I am.

H.- The thing that moves me is that object on the horizon that keeps showing up, not the love of another. This was given to me by my Mother.

My Mama said "Look when you were born into the world, you weren't born with a twin. So, remember this; The love that is going to secure you through life is the love that you offer yourself, not the love of another that could come and go."

I love women. Every woman I've been with I loved. I love them now. But I do not depend on their love. You ask about the young lady with us. She said, "She loves me." She's 25 and I'm 82. I'm supposed

to be jumping for joy. Not so, my eyes are on the prize, which is Africa. I don't believe I would ever feel as comfortable as I would like to feel. If I do not accomplish the goals that I'm pursuing.

I've been married four times. I came home and found my wife with another man. I didn't feel bad. I feel good. My Grandpa always said, "Get another one quick." It's beautiful. These are the things that we need to cultivate, not the dependency of another. Why should you be depending on me for love? Depend on yourself, that love would never die. But if you depend on me, why would you want to do that? Why would I even want love from a woman? When one day she tells you "I don't love you anymore." Well, that's fine, keep on stepping. But my friend John, he didn't do that, he killed himself. We were on a cruise ship. I was a merchant seaman. He killed himself. He jumped over the side of the ship over the thing called "love." So, you love the word "love" we need to examine that.

Q.- What is that goal that you want to accomplish?

H.- Heighten Africa.

Q.- I understand that you had some disappointments and frustrations in dealing with the African government and African leaders. That after you presented your body of work and the different people you have healed and many countries in Africa are so desperately in need of a way to address. Just start with AIDS. But for the most part, they rejected your approach.

H.- Of course, and they were right to reject me! Not only Africa. I quit my job as an engineer to go to Dominica. I went to Dominica and I was happy. Beautiful Island, beautiful people. People were cured of blindness, diabetes, and a whole lot of other stuff.

Q.- You said people were cured?

H.- Yes, while I was there and Mrs. Eugenia Charles said "You got to go."

I said, "But Mrs. Charles, I'm doing a service here."

"Look, you got to go!"

OK, she kicks me out. Me and my crazy self, I went to South Africa under the leadership of Mr. Nelson Mandela. I went to the board of health and presented what I've done. I showed them all of my documents and diagnostic sheets. AIDS is devastating in South Africa. So, I thought because I can do this job, that I would be received with love, that's all. All I wanted was love, right! Understood?

Mandela said get out of here! Nelson Mandela! Wait another one, Mr. Robert Mugabe from Zimbabwe. I got to Zimbabwe. I took all these boxes of the compound. Oh, I was happy. I was going to do some work in Africa. He said get out! I said "Wow what's wrong with me? What have I done wrong?"

But when I look at it carefully. The Africans were right to reject me. Every African country is 100% right.

Q.- Why do you say that?

H.- They are right because the African people were totally unaware that what they are eating is undermining their struggle. Undermining their own existence. Africa is eating starch and blood. Starch and blood. Now, let's take that to the laboratory and see if there's food there. Not there! no food.

Q.- You mentioned earlier in the Dominican Republic that you cured blindness. The issue of retinitis pigmentosa is certainly one form of blindness. What in the world is it? Because on the surface, these positions that you take and the claims that you make are what anybody would say is "Unbelievable" however those who suffer from these maladies want to have a form of hope. So, I would ask you to work with me here and walk me through meeting someone who's blind and what you do to or with them to give them sight.

H.- You know when I was kicked out of Dominica, I didn't know where to go. My wife said to me, "Then go to Sin Cloy." I didn't know anything about Sin Cloy, but I went. When I got to Sin Cloy everybody in Sin Cloy just hated me. They found the light in hating me. Because I was making these statements and it upset people.

I'm broke now. I just quit my job a year ago and I don't know what to do. Because the woman kicked me out of Dominica and I spent all my money on things and a house. So, while I was in Sin Cloy things were looking bad. I had to call my brother to borrow some money. One day my wife said to me "I want you to go to the supermarket and buy some food for the children." We got our last $200. I went to the supermarket and on my way out of the register, someone in the back of the line called my name.

"I wanted to thank you for curing my husband."

I said, "Ma'am, I have not cured anyone in Sin Cloy."

"No, you cured him in Dominica, he was blind."

I said, "Wait, the only blind man that I have ever treated and cured lives in Los Angeles, Mr. Frederick."

She said, "No, you cured my husband."

I said, "How can I have cured your husband and I didn't know it?"

She said "The policeman that used to come to pick up the remedy and he would take it to my husband didn't tell you what he had. My husband was blind for 11 years."

So, you're asking me how can I cure a blind man without seeing him? Well, let me say this. The philosophy of Europe claimed that when you're blind, something is wrong with your eyes. The philosopher from Africa said, or the understanding of Africa, NOT SO! When you're blind something is wrong with your stomach. You clean the intestine, then your eyes start to clear up. This is the science that is unknown to the world, but it works for me.

The other day a young man named Mr. G, a beautiful young man. The brilliant young man said to me "My sister had lupus." Who cures lupus? Nobody. Three months later his sister doesn't have lupus anymore. I was happy that I had cured her from lupus. Because I wanted this one to work because this is my friend Mr. G.

Q.- I'm putting some focus on the issue of retinitis pigmentosa. Because I know someone very close. He's legally blind now. What is something you do that he should try?

H.- Well, clean the body out again. Cleansing again. All they have to do is call my office and they will send him a package. An eyewash and a stomach wash and immediately he will see the result, immediately!

As you said earlier, "It sounds fantastic." But if you're traveling to Africa your compass better says 90*, not 270* you're going west, am I right? So, if you're traveling on a route you better put your compass on the right course. All these years we have been following medical science. They say that disease is what? Germs, viruses, bacteria? I said "NO! It's the food that you eat. The food better be consistent with you."

Gorillas do not eat Polar bear food. But if the Gorilla ever makes the mistake and puts it in his mouth, the food of the Polar bear. He too would find the disease that we are finding ourselves with. It happened right here in New York, in the zoo. Gorillas in the zoo got diabetes. Not in the forest.

Chapter 6

Electric Food for the Electric Body

Q.- What is melanin? And what is carbon? Can you please describe those?

H.- Melanin is not a mineral. Melanin is a word that was used to describe a certain geological function. But in that particular identification or category or thing, melanin is the European identification of what they think activates those neurons in our body that make us Black. But when you break down our body, our biological structure into what we would have to put it in. Which is biochemistry. Melanin has no place. It is not to be found. What is found in the body that is attributed to melanin is carbon. Carbon not only determines the quality of life in Black folks. **But Carbon determines the quality of life in every living plant that exists.** If carbon is absent, there's no life.

So, "Melanin." What is it? I don't know. White folks also talk about protein. What is protein? They say "It's one of the nineteen amino acids, the building blocks of life." But I know for a fact that's not a true statement. Because if protein is the building block of life, what happened to the gorilla that lived up to 180 years without eating anything that contains protein? Unless they're going to say that the plants contain protein too. They're always saying things. We have no laboratory to investigate those things. Then we have to swallow it's line, hook, and sinker.

Mrs. Francis mentioned melanin and I asked her "What are those things?" And I know she cannot adequately answer the question. Because she was trained by someone European. So, when you are trained by European and are told these things, you have to regurgitate them back. But they are completely in error. So, we have to be careful. Remember it is like a brother recommends that you use Comfrey for your bones. That is in the books from Europeans' philosophical base. But if you look at Comfrey, it contains starch. Again, another European philosophy. Melanin falls under the same category. It's a belief, not reality.

I was told in Washington DC that I was violating one of the most sacred codes or laws of nutrition when I deprived Akeela Strough of protein.

So, I ask Dr. Steinberg and Dr. Glut at Georgetown Pediatric Hospital. "Did you give her protein five times a day? You did. Was she under your cure for 2 years? Yes. Now that she does not receive those things you call "protein", she no longer has sickle cell anemia. So where is the validity in this thing we call "protein"? Is it equity? Or is it a deficit?

We don't know! When I embarked on the journey of healing many were asking me; "Why are you so concerned with the scientific aspect of these things?"

I had to because my challenge would be from a scientific base. If I didn't understand science then I would be lost and they would gain momentum when they should not.

So, I said "It is necessary, but not to heal. To heal it is necessary to understand the scientific aspect of it. But you must understand the herb that corresponds with the disease that is manifesting. The only way you can do that in the Western World and to prove that and would be respected as someone that could be of usefulness. Is to enhance oneself with the words that describe certain things and that's the science of biochemistry."

So, I decide to go into the scientific understanding of these things we call "herbs." What we found is that there are things on the planet that assimilate and can be of usefulness. Say that substance is electrical and the only electric substance on the planet is natural plants. Not Comfrey, Goldenseal, Peppermint, Aloe Vera, and the rest of hybrid plants. How many brothers and sisters or anyone in the world qualifies to offer a challenge? When we have nothing to test that, we are given it for validity.

No, I do not subscribe to melanin or Comfrey. So again, we have to go back to the drawing board. The Usha Research disregards the word melanin. For instance, if melanin determines life, why is it that when people come to us with nerve problems or with energy problems, we give them a substance known as "iron" which is a mineral. And strengthen that iron with carbon, hydrogen, and oxygen, the C.H.O chain of life. Carbon, hydrogen, and oxygen, melanin has no place in that biochemical structure. So, I'm extremely sorry.

Q.- What makes a difference between black and white? Why is one person of color and another is not?

H.- Well again, we can easily explain that position. Carbon is the determining factor for your color. The concentration of carbon determines the color black. The higher concentration of carbon, the greater the color black expresses. It is carbon, nothing else.

Q.- Please explain to the people the word "electric/electricity" and how it pertains to its necessity or boundaries within the body structure.

H.- Now that was the best question that could have been asked. Why? Because it's something useful in our biological structure. It must be electrical and the only substance that is electrical are those substances that come from the forest or the jungle. Because the molecular structure is complete, not broken. If something is made by mother nature, one can easily use their common sense and see that this stuff is natural and is complete. But if something is made in a laboratory, common sense again shows us it could not be of usefulness.

For instance, iron has to have 1000 electrons per atom, calcium has 9000 and opium has a specific amount. So, it goes to the whole. It expresses itself differently. **Because that is necessary to maintain continuity to maintain the individuality of each plant.**

The bone is calcium, not blood, blood is iron. Now we go back to the question of melanin. Would it be intelligent to ask one of the promoters of melanin "What is the electromagnetic structure of melanin? What is the amount of electrons per atom that represents this thing we called melanin?" Why do we ask the question? Because it is necessary. We want to know if this thing is electrical. Well, if it is electrical, it has to have a definite amount of electrons per atom representing that particular thing.

Q.- Let me ask you another question on that same subject. Let's say the generator that gives us electricity here in our city was cut off and we wanted to get more electricity. What will we do? Will we stick one end to the ground? How would that work?

H.- Stick what into the ground

Q.- A wire.

H.- No, what produces electricity?

Q.- Electron.

H.- No way! I was an electrician. I am an engineer. I worked in what you call a steam generating plant. I have a degree. I have a license in what is known as thermal dynamic. We are dealing with physics now. The only thing that produces electricity is the friction between copper and carbon. That could be seen in your automobile. Take out your generator and see what it has inside. It has

copper wheels and carbon brushes that touch against it when it turns. Here's an example: this is the copper wheel in the generator plant that produces electricity for this room. It is spinning at 90 revolutions per minute. Rubbing against this copper wheel there are carbon brushes. And this is what you see; the spinning of the copper wheel against the carbon brush creates friction. The friction is called resonant. Resonant is electricity. Not electrons. Resonate! The resonance produces electrons, not before. So now if electricity is produced by the friction of carbon and copper then where do we go in the human body and find the organs that produce electricity?

We find that in the brain, it is the center of the motor. The nervous system is the conduit that carries electricity to various points of the body to cause motion. Now should we ask "What is the composition of the brain?" It is made up of carbon and copper. The pineal gland is carbon and the cerebral cortex is copper. We don't only find it in human beings. We find it in the eel of Brazil that produces electricity to kill its prey. When you open the eel all you find is carbon and copper, no melanin.

Q.- Does everyone have a pineal gland?

H.- If you have no pineal gland you would not be alive. There would be no motion, it's impossible. Every race has a pineal gland. Not every race has a thyroid gland. The thyroid gland regulates sex. It also maintains energy. The thyroid gland keeps you childlike, non-aggressive. But in some races the thyroid gland disappears at the age of 8, then one becomes violent in one's movement. Now if the thyroid gland disappears in some races at age 8 specifically Caucasian. What helps one to retain the thyroid gland within biology? The presence of what? **Carbon,** thank you.

Q.- What you're saying is that due to the way medical students study medicine here and around the world. They don't understand the human's electric body?

H.- **Well, if we're talking about understanding. What do they understand? Because the question needs to be asked. Remember, the time for common sense has risen and arrived. What do they understand? Don't be afraid. We need to ask these questions. What do they understand? No cure for the common cold, no cure for diabetes, no cure for cancer, lupus, AIDS, sickle cell anemia, blindness, or any other disease. Well, if the physician clearly shows us that there is no cure for any disease. What do they understand?**

So, we have to throw away that understanding and that premise out the window. Everything that comes from the physician has to be thrown away in the trash. Because there's no positive outcome. What have they done as far as usefulness in reference to pathology? What have they reversed? Nothing! So why should their words be the authority? We can't use them as some level of thinking, or development, or seeing. No, we can't do that, they don't have it and they showed us. How old is the medicine that they are practicing today? It is 265 years old.

It starts with Bombastic Bonhomminhym only because he was prejudiced. When he found out that Hippocrates went to Africa to learn his craft, the fact of the matter is that Mr. Hippocrates 2000 years ago used herbs to cure every disease known to man. If Mr. Hippocrates used herbs to cure every disease known to man, then 2000 years later why aren't we doing so? Because the healer has been educated. And the substances he uses are artificial and he is totally unaware of that. Why? Because he learns his craft from an armchair position. They call that armchair research, not field research. And it's very important to know your herbs from a field position. Why?

Because in 1973, I sent Mr. Adam to St. John's herb store. I ask him to buy me a pound of Bugleweed. Why did I want Bugleweed? Because someone came to me with a very bad heart problem.

They call it "Mitral Stenosis" the weakening of the heart muscle.

I said, "Buy me a pound of Bugleweed because I have to address a particular disease."

When Adam came back with the Bugleweed. I opened the bag and said, "Where is the Bugleweed?"

He said, "In the bag."

I said "No, that is not Bugleweed."

He said, "What is it?"

I said, "That's Blue Vervain."

"How do you know?"

I said "I tasted it and it was sweet and I can look at it. That's how I can tell."

I didn't learn herbs by reading a book. That's what the herbalist does in New York and the United States.

I said, "Take me back to the store."

So, he took me to the store and there was a young lady, which was Black said to me "Well, how do you know that this is not Bugleweed? My boss has been selling herbs for 25 years."

I said "Young lady your boss can be selling herbs for 125 years. This isn't Bugleweed, call your boss."

The boss came "What's the problem?"

I said "I don't think there's a problem. There's never been a problem with me. I don't have those things. But you sold me one thing, it was supposed to be another."

"How do you know?"

I know this is not Bugleweed. Bugleweed is bitter as gall and this is sweet. Bugleweed has little balls on the plant. Every inch has a little ball. This has no balls.

I said "Can you please go and see if the bag that was sent to you that was labeled Blue Vervain can be the Bugleweed"

And she goes inside and guesses what happened? The bag was mislabeled and she apologized.

But if I had not known about the herbs and did not properly learn about them, she would have misled me. I could give it to anybody in New York and they would say this and that and they would not know. Because the very herbalist is recommending carrot juice. When I came to New York 15 years ago, one of them was telling their recipient to drink carrot juice. Then tell their recipient to take Goldenseal. Well, when you do such a thing, you're showing the world that you don't know what you are doing.

This happened to me when I went to the W.L.I.B. radio station. I told the audience at W.L.I.B. that carrots were artificial. They all denied me. A year later when NOVA came out with the program. Not only was it artificial. They showed that it was made by crossing Queen Anne Lace and the Wild Yam. You do not mix herbs unless they belong to the same balance. What do I mean by that? I mean this; in the kingdom of life, a Yaeko plant known as Queen Anne Lace can only pollinate with another Queen Anne Lace. Why? Because the pollen carries the same amount of balance as the other and through that process we know as "chemical affinity", they join.

Now, there is another mixture that we are totally unaware of besides the natural one which is chemical affinity. The other one is a mechanical mixture. What is a mechanical mixture? A mechanical mixture is when you cut a sliver in a plant like Queen Anne Lace, and you cut a sliver in another plant and you take out the heart of the stem and you put it inside of Queen Anne Lace and then tape it, that is hybridization.

Black people know nothing about this. Now, this plant produces something other than what it was supposed to originally. Because now you're writing Queen Anne Lace with Wild Yam. You don't get Queen Anne Lace or the Wild Yam. You get what? A carrot. They went further to show that it was made in Holland and a little before that article came out. I had returned to the drawing board to find that this carrot is artificial. I knew it was artificial, why? Because it doesn't produce seeds to produce itself. So, I knew it was artificial and besides that, it contains starch.

When I went back to do my research, guess what I found? That Germans made the lamb and barley. I see why the Arabs are so indebted to Germany. Because the Germans made the Arab's food. The Arabs had no food you know. Arabia never had food. Arabia doesn't have food now. Nowhere inside Arabia, you find natural food. Everything the Arabs eat, the very Quran that they read came out of Germany. Also, their food. If the Germans remove the food from the Arabs, they starve to death. This is nasty, isn't it? Oh yes, it is. It is treacherous you see. Many of us Blacks hold the Arabs supreme. Not in my book. Because how can someone eat unnatural food and be smart? When the very food that you eat influences the brain to allow you to think and if you eat the wrong things, that again is common sense.

If you take a diesel automobile and put in gasoline. What happens? It cannot run. The human body responds in the same way. The Black race never really had anyone to show us what we should or should not eat. The only man that came was the messenger, our honorable Elijah Mohammed. The only man that said, "Stay away from the pork." And when I sat and ate with the messenger in his house on 3837 South Woodlawn Ave in Chicago. The messenger personally told me and brother Nance from New Orleans that we should not be eating meat at all. We should not be eating anything on this menu. Because it is poisonous to us. But if he, the messenger of Allah, Elijah Mohammed had told the Black race of the United States to stop everything. Who would listen then? So, he had to, he couldn't cold turkey us. He was very intelligent. He removed the pork and many other little things.

We have been conditioned. They have made us addicts. Which Black person in America eats food that is consistent with their African ancestors? None.

Then we go to the Maya Honduras where I was born. That's a Latin American country. I asked a question to one of the guides. They guide tourists in and out of the ruins and explain about the Maya.

I asked him "Sir do you mind if I ask you a question?"

He said "No."

"What did the Maya eat?"

A lady that was part of the tour in the group jumped up and said "Corn of course!"

The man looked at me, I looked at the lady and he said "Lady, if the Maya ate corn, this man here would not have asked that question. He would have known that."

So, there's something about that corn that we have to question. Then he turned back to me and he said "What did they eat?"

I said "I could begin with Teo Sinti, the Caploata, the Chipiling these are natural greens that grow in the forest of Honduras. The Teo Sinti is a plant that produces a kernel that looks like corn. But the difference is, it is non-starch. They make the tamale from the Teo Senti and they mix the Chipilini which is green and they make these tamales and they still do it in Santa Rosa DE Copán. And when you all come to Honduras, I will introduce you guys to these tamales that are all-natural."

The Maya did not eat corn, rice, beans, chicken, egg, pork, or cow. Why? Because these things did not exist in Honduras before Christopher Columbus came. They only ate those things that were natural. But the guide knew that he didn't know what the Maya ate. How many Africans in Africa know what their ancestors ate? They don't know. What do Africans eat today? Rice, that's all they have and rice is poison. Not only is it starch, but it also converts into carbonic acid and it contains cyanide.

Q.- How about Asian people? They eat it every day.

H.- Well, what about them? Because they eat it every day. Are they the healthiest people in the world? You never see a Japanese or Chinese walk straight. His spine could just not hold up straight. He always walks with a drop in his spine. He just can't do it. He eats nothing but starch. The Chinese should give credit and a lot of credit to the Italian that went down there, Marco Polo. Because at least he took down there the wheat kernels so that they can make their noodles. Before Marco Polo, the Chinese couldn't make noodles.

Q.- What about the Buddhist monks or Confucius were they still eating the same poison?

H.- What else do they have to eat? There's only one man that came out of China that understood. That was Dr. Li Ching-Yuen. Dr. Li didn't eat anything that didn't grow in the ground. No, he didn't. He just didn't do that and Dr. Li according to history lived 256 years. He died here in New York, or it was recorded in New York, he died in China. He was a China man that I respect.

Like when I went to India, I talked to Raja Gorchapachari. He's a friend of mine that lives in Kolkata. He looked at all the Indians and he said "They're all dead."

I said, "Why?"

"Look at what they eat."

I said the same about Africans. That's why there isn't one African leader that I respect. I can't respect any African leader. Because I know his head is confounded. Why? "Because look at what he eats."

Q.- Is fish good?

H.- Fish rots in the intestine.

Q.- That's where the worm goes?

H.- Exactly right. Anything that walks, crawls, swims, flies or that has a head, should not enter my system.

Q.- With this New Age Movement and all herbalists and writers. Do you recommend any of these books or teachings? Now that a lot of people are going back to nature and heading to these herbology stores with all the varieties of products. Our people are still confused because of a lack of correct information or misinformation. Can you direct us on a path and what things we need to stay away from?

H.- Head to the forest with someone that came from the forest, that we have not had! Because some of the best advisers in the United States, counselors, nutritionists, and doctors train our brother by the name of Dick Gregory. Did he recommend the Bohemia diet? The answer is "Yes" and what does the Bohemia diet consist of as a base? Soybean. And didn't Mr. George Washington Carver make plastic out of soybean? Yes. So how could he give us the Bohemia diet that is soybean base in the name of nutrition? But we cannot blame Dick Gregory cause he's our brother. I know he loves us and we love him. But he was ill-trained. The students can only regurgitate what was learned from the teacher. If the teacher is poorly educated then the student likewise.

Q.- Can you share more knowledge about the carrot and different potatoes? Sweet potato is ok but the white potato we should stay from?

H.- I didn't say sweet potato was alright: that was made, too.

Q.- Is there a certain kind?

H.- **The Red Potato and the Red Rose that was found in Lake Titicaca in Peru, that is where the Irish people became acquainted and took it back to Ireland. Remember, the Irish people were the first to go to Peru. They did a lot of things in Peru. When they found this potato. They took it back to Ireland and they began the hybridization of the potatoes and got what you call the Russet Potato...the Red Rose... But the natural potato looks like the Red Rose. I would recommend that you eat that because it's the first generation away from the mother... from the base which came from Lake Titicaca. But not the sweet potato: a sweet potato has such a high concentration of nitrogen that it would really cause havoc in the system.**

This book is needed. We have been misled by the foreigners... that are not part of our race, but dictate to us and tell us what we should or should not eat. But we were also hoodwinked by our brothers, who were trained by those people. The Gorilla does not eat the food of a lion. So, we can't eat Chinese food or Caucasian food. We're not Caucasian, we're not Chinese. We are Black and what does that mean? I use

the word Black and I use it too loosely. Because I don't like the word.

Q.- What's a good word?

H.- I don't know.

Q.- The shadows?

H.- No! I am, you call me negro, you call me nigga, you call me color boy, you call me black, you call me African. I'm not an African because the continent was not called Africa until the white man called it Africa, so what are we?

Q.- Planetariums? I want to ask about spirulina and wheatgrass.

H.- Spirulina, where does Spirulina grow? It's a hybrid. What about the wheatgrass? Hybrid. When I was in my brandish stages... I must admit, it was later than that because I was in New York practicing this thing already. I was using wheat to produce wheatgrass to be juice and here I go with this little cup of wheatgrass juice. I have the best chlorophyll in the world.

Man... a little lady 94 years of age named Mrs. Holloman said "You're out of your mind! You're not going to recommend that to yourself or no one else."

"Why Mrs. Holloman?"

"Because this stuff is poison."

"Wheatgrass juice?"

Wait, just a minute is wheat natural?

I said, "No." The fennel is natural, the teff is natural. But not the wheat. You make bread out of fennel. You make bread out of teff. Which is the brown Injera from Ethiopia. Which is made out of teff. But as far as wheat goes, oh we have to remember the Amaranth which is natural.

But this thing we called wheat? Definitely made in Europe. When we grow this kernel and we squeeze it. We get sugar and starch. So, my brain tells me don't use it anymore. What do you use? Sprout of something natural. So, I went and got some Amaranth. Amaranth Seed can be acquired right in Brooklyn, it grows all over the place.

For instance, if you take the little wheatgrass seeds and put them on the bed right now and cover it with soil. In 21 days, the wheatgrass sprouts. But the Amaranth will not sprout in 21 days. Why? The Amaranth only sprouts once a year, in the Spring. Because it is natural.

So, I was angry because the Amaranth did not sprout. Then the Amaranth laughed at me and said "You want me to sprout along with something hybrid? I'm very sorry I only sprout once a year. The product I produce is food." And when the Amaranth sprout came, oh... I was high for about 3 months. I was on this high, this energy. Because the molecular structure is complete and therefore it deems that this stuff is electrical. If the molecular structure is incomplete "meaning it's a hybrid plant" it cannot be electrical.

If a man can make a substance in a laboratory such as vitamin C, vitamin D, vitamin B12, zinc all this stuff. Wait just a minute! How could you make it in a laboratory a substance that would help me biologically or physiologically? If you can do that and if you can really do that, then you're GOD. Only nature or GOD can make something electrical. No man can do that!

I will give a simple example. On the planet, minerals are expressed in two forms. One phosphate and one oxide meaning what?

There are 102 minerals... We begin with gold, silver, iron, phosphorus, magnesium, they come in the form of a rock. But that rock also has a plant that is representative of that mineral. A plant that contains gold...GOLD!? Why should it be so difficult for you to understand that? Don't you take Burdock for iron? What's the difference between iron and gold? They're both minerals. But now you have them in a plant form. Why a plant form? Because the plant is sending its roots in the soil and converts that solid rock into a liquid digestible substance. The scientist calls that the process of conversion iontophoresis. Iontophoresis can only be accomplished by a plant, not a laboratory. You can't take a piece of rock that is iron into a laboratory and get liquid from it that's going to be digestible, and it's non-electrical. The plant makes it electrical. When you drink it, it's pre-digestive and It's electrical!

So that no one misled you. The minerals that the body needs cannot be found in any health food store.

No vitamin C, vitamin B, or vitamin A. The body is not made up of any alphabetical order. It is made up of minerals. When those minerals have been depleted by the presence of disease, a disease is in suit. So, you have to replace them in a natural form.

In the form of a rock or plant? A plant because it is alive and it's electrical. How can you feed an electric body dead food? You just can't do that. That's not consistency.

Q.- So when a person goes to the hospital and they're given so-called "treatments." We know when someone is treated for something it has nothing to do with the cure. When you have something like the American Cancer Society, they mention nothing about curing people. They are just a cancer society. In which they study, study some more, get some more money and keep studying. But never finding the cure. When the cure is something natural in the ground and the body can heal itself eventually. But yet what they do is they propagandize a natural disease and made a big multibillion-dollar industry because of it.

H.- Of course, and they are right 100%. If I was a Caucasian, defending my people and my economic position. Do you think I would undermine that position? By telling the world here's a Black man that has cured diabetes, sickle cell anemia, leukemia. Then what's going to happen to his pharmaceutical laboratory? Why should we be concerned with the American Medical Association?

Q.- What's the name of the organization that's going around spreading AIDS on our folks?

H.- The WORLD HEALTH ORGANIZATION.

Q.- That's right! The W.H.O, what do you think about them?

H.- I was in Washington, DC in 1982. This brother is a doctor, who worked for the W.H.O. They told me they threw in the towel 20 years ago. That they knew that there was no cure for any disease. They never had one. I mean the physicians didn't learn to cure anyone. Their discipline just doesn't house that. So again, we should not be bringing them up, because of no positive outcome.

Q.- The only thing is they are killing our folks over there in Africa. When are they going to learn?

H.- They are killing our folks in Africa?

Q.- Yeah, they're all coming up with AIDS. Where did they get AIDS from?

H. But the Africans need to be killed. I mean coming from me to say that his family needs to be killed. But that's a FACT! The Africans have turned their back on their Mother. In fact, Africans have never regarded a Black Woman as being equal to a male. So, when you abandon your position you need to pay the dire consequences. When you abandon your mother and I'm not talking only about our biological Mother. I'm talking about that greater Mother, Africa! They change Africa. They made an exchange for Europe. In Africa, they deserve to die. Everyone that dies deserves to die or else they would not be dying.

Q.- I think you're right.

H.- I know I'm right, they wouldn't be dying now.

Q.- The organization has got to have someone with some sense.

H.- And it's not there. That's why I said, "I would prefer to take a shoeshine boy from New York and put him in the Presidency in Africa or any country and he would do a better job than those that are there now." Because common sense just steps out the window. The Africans don't eat anything that came from their ancestors. What do they eat? They eat rice and sweet potatoes. Have you ever tried to put a salad bowl beside an African before he eats, to see if he's going to eat the salad?

Q.- AIDS seems to be plaguing us at this moment. What is your take on it?

H.- Well, this book that you raised if you notice carefully, it reads "AIDS, the good news is HIV doesn't cause it." And under here it said Peter Duesberg. This man was the only man that made a statement that was in my favor when I was going through my litigation. This man was a White man. Peter Duesberg said that AIDS was not the result of a virus and I agree with him. I have yet to have a brother physician or otherwise, that openly agrees with me. Peter Duesberg did, he was at the University of Berkeley California. Duesberg is a microbiologist. They removed his grants and kicked him out.

That was ok. Now they have an organization known as HEAL. He's heading that and it's all over the world.

In fact, someone wants me to get in touch with them because they were looking for me. But this man was right, AIDS was a long time coming. Another doctor by the name of Stucker. He was a protégé of Duesberg. He said that when they went to Africa and inoculated the Africans with smallpox and polio vaccine. That was the beginning of AIDS.

Dr. Love, Dr. Rashad, and Dr. Prince sat in a counseling room. Mr. Valentine was one of them who kicked me out of New York. Our brother that cured AIDS and you want to kick him out of New York? Mr. Valentine did that, Mr. Valentine turned against me!

Which one of them is interested in the cure for Black folks? Say for instance ten of us set out to do research and nine fail. The brother over here Mr. Simon found the cure for AIDS. What should the nine of us do? Come to you cause you're the reason they found it. Mr. Valentine, Dr. Love Khania, Dr. Prince, Doctor all of them said GOOD LUCK! I said thank you very much.

Q.- What about Dr. Barbara Justice?

H.- She doesn't like me and she is right. She should not like me and I hope she reads this book. Because I love this idea that Barbara Justice doesn't like him. She has to live with that hate herself and I hope that hate doesn't last too long, hahaha.

Q.- Years ago my father Prof. George Simmons got out of the hospital and was feeling really weak, this was 1988. He did not know what to do. So, his friend sends him to Dr.

Barbara Justice and she looked at him and said, "All you can do is just pray and wait to die." So, what happened was a few of my father's friends took me to see you "The Healer" over here. And my father, if you recall the first time you met him. I took him to your office. He told you all these problems that he was this and that. He said you didn't look at him. You were too busy reading something. You told him don't worry about it, you'll be OK in a couple of weeks or a couple of months. You said he'll be back teaching without much of a problem. Long and behold, my father did what you told him to do and he was back teaching around that time frame. He's been running around now down in Honduras at your institute. He went down there with all these different maladies such as diabetes, prostate cancer, high blood pressure, and a whole bunch of things. He said within 2 days of being down there, he was ready to run an Olympic event.

H.- And he did! His sugar was down to 93 and his toe that was supposed to be amputated no longer had to be amputated. His hair was growing back, did he tell you? His hair was growing back before it was falling out. The village that I was talking about is here (showing a picture). This is the village. We see the tanks with the thermal water. This is the Usha Village in Central America and you see these tanks house the water. The thermal water contains a PH of 8.8. It is not like what they have in other places. I've heard that there's a hot spring in Cottonwood, Alabama. We don't have hot springs in Honduras. We have a thermal spring and the difference from a thermal spring is that the thermal spring is reciprocated by volcanic activity. Which means the water has a high concentration of sulfur and phosphorus. Not so for a

hot spring. A hot spring is reciprocated through a bed of zeolite that's under the ground that's boiling the water. That does not make it thermal.

Q.- So what makes the difference?

H.- One has sulfur, phosphorus, and oxygen in large amounts.

Q.- Which means what to the body?

H.- It means that the body is receiving a large amount of hydrogen ion concentration that relaxes the body immediately. It plays a very good role in the central nervous system. Stress is gone immediately after entering the water and that was the first thing that I did for the professor after he got there. I said "Before you eat or go to sleep. You go down there and take a bath." We took him down there and he took a bath, the next day he was rejoicing.

Q.- And what happens when stress is relieved from the body?

H.- The body begins to normalize itself. The hormones begin to take the messes where they need to go. When there's a nerve condition, hormones tend to contract or retain or they don't do their work. Because they are held back. Bell's Palsy is one. Bell's Palsy is caused by an emotional reaction. It pulls the muscle to one side and when the person relaxes, again the muscles relax.

Q.- So the remedy in Bell's Palsy is to get into a non stressful or relaxed state. By taking one of these baths?

H.- That's right, it's not one of these baths. You take baths twice a day and then you take internal therapy. Which is what? The Pavana, the Cordoncillo Negro, the Si-Press, and yes, my most favorite the Draco. These are the plants you'll never hear in the American standard pharmaceutical corporation. You don't even hear these herbs in the mouth of the herbalist in Honduras or the United States for that matter. Even Honduras when asked for those herbs that are of use and they don't even know them. Because they are too busy reading herbal books. Those herbs are not in the herbal books.

Q.- I wish very much that you can meet Dr. Anthony Handoff. He was an ethnobotanist. He went to school and got there...

H.- I don't think I want to meet the brother now. It's not that I don't want to meet my brother. But I can't exchange or even entertain someone that has been educated. Remember what I said, the reason why the healers are not healing today is that they have been educated. You want to hear a beautiful one above all else.

Dr. David Iansu is a member of the Smithsonian Institution. There's a program out known as "East meets West." Meaning African or Eastern Medicine against Western. They begin to show where this

African in Africa took some herbs and put them on this lady's head because she was crazy. The African Healer took a knife and opened her skull. She took some smoke and blew smoke around the woman. While Dr. David Iansu was talking about the herbs of his people. He's from Ghana and he's a member of the Smithsonian Institution. Dr. David Iansu is the brother that's looking for a cure for leukemia using the Rosy Periwinkle. Well, I don't know how Dr. David Iansu expects to derive from the Rosy Periwinkle cure for leukemia. When the Rosy Periwinkle is also an acid plant and as for leukemia. We have cured leukemia long before Dr. Iansu even dreamed of coming on with Rosy Periwinkle.

But we go back again and we find at the end of the program East meets West. Which is approximately a 25 years old program. Showing the comparison of Western Medicine against Ancient Medicine and guess who wins every time? Western Medicine, the Allopathic. In the end, Dr. David Iansu and his colleague said "Well you can clearly see that traditional medicine is alright. You know but it falls short. Because you can't really measure the dosage for consistency. So modern medicine is by far the best" and they end the program.

I said, "That was so beautiful." But I knew that a day would come in which the philosophy that Dr. David Iansu is supporting and the African Bio-Mineral Balance would come face to face one day and it happened. Dr. David Iansu called me and said, "I heard about your work on leukemia. But we are looking for the cure for leukemia with the Rosy Periwinkle."

I said, "Dr. David Iansu, we already cure leukemia. You can just squash that and just go to something else."

That was 12 years ago when I told him that, 12 years ago...

Black America and still now does not show the interest in our health and healing the way that we should. All of the healers in New York, I don't recall their names but they all read books. If I take Dr. Phil Valentine and Dr. Love and Dr... into the forest. They wouldn't know a natural herb from an artificial one. But we can't blame the brothers. They were ill-prepared because they were prepared by a Caucasian.

Q.- On the subject of that, you don't want to meet up with a particular individual. This is for clarification. It's not that you don't want to meet them. But based on your experience of dealing with individuals who come with certain credentials or papers from the establishment of the system schools. That you know that there's a great difficulty in a back and forth between the dialogue.

H.- My response is this; we are told by our brother that the system wants us to meet an ethnobotanist. What do they cure?

Q.- Researches different plants.

H.- I'm only asking what do they cure? Research is 150 years old. We can research and research and research and research! We want a cure! We don't want

to research. And just research, research, research.
What does he cure?

Q.- Well he has different plants. He tells you that you
can take that and that will cure.

H.- Wait, hold it. How does he know that? What
does he cure?

Q.- He's from Africa and he was taught by his father
and grandfather so forth and he said he's only using plants
from the homeland.

H.- You mine if I ask the question again? What
does he cure?

Q.- Any disease.

H.- Does he cure AIDS?

Q.- I'm sure he does.

H.- Well that's good. If he cured AIDS. I'm the only
individual that have diagnostic sheets showing from five
different laboratories around the world showing that he
has been cured of AIDS. I don't say it. I got diagnostic
sheets and that's important. Who else has those
diagnostic sheets? Thank you. So, I can't lend myself to
someone that said that he does. Where's the proof?

Q.- I used to go to a few meetings and I was sponsored
by Burrow Welcome European Allopathic Medical
Establishment and then they formed an organization

known as HEAL. Which people like Peter Duesburg support. That group and HEAL, of course, I'm sure they can find you. Because many of us loved you. When you left us. We just felt so abandoned.

H.- Why can't Black people find me instead of HEAL? That's more important to me than HEAL. Black people are not interested in their health right now. But Latin America is interested in their health right now. We have a gatherer of people taking to the forest of Brazil, Peru, Chile, Honduras, Guatemala, Salvador who's right now researching the forest. None of them are Americans and none of them are Blacks. Why? We talk and we talk and we talk and we research and we research and we research and we spend all of life researching and diseases are all running rapidly.

Q.- But we have to start somewhere. We have to begin with research.

H.- That's a solvable position, that's a very solvable position.

Q.- You gotta start somewhere.

H.- How long is research? My research took me two years and now we cure sickle cell anemia. We cure AIDS and we cure blindness. But these other men have 25 years under their belt and what do they cure?

Q.- You're absolutely right. But you have to start with research in the beginning.

H.- I call it research because my Grandmother was the one that did it. See, my Grandmother was a healer and she didn't go to school.

Q.- Research can be like running a relay race. Somebody else can cover the grounds and you'll know about it. Then you pick up the race from where they are.

H.- But if the race started off heading in the wrong direction, you lose. The finish line is receding faster than you can run.

Q.- Hahaha, what happens is you pass the baton and there's no finish line.

H.- You're right. It's behind you. So, I don't want to hear about research. If I was in South America, people don't bring to me these questions. Not in South America. I live in South America. They say "We know of no one that cured the diseases you have cured. So, you have the blessing of our country. Honduras has given you all the privilege to practice your craft regardless of what the world says."

"You can go to Africa."

I said "No"

"But you're an African by heritage."

"But I can't go there, they kicked me out."

Q.- So the research need can be attributed in part to the conditioning that many of us have been taught to say.

"Well, where's your research?" As you pointed out to be apathetic.

H.- "What have you done?" not "What have you researched?" What have you done! That's Latin America. But that in America, it's arrogant. But we are arrogant! As Professor George Simmons said, that I am considered an arrogant individual. Yes, not only you were arrogant, everybody in Honduras is arrogant. You have been independent since 1824. You have earned your position to be arrogant. Especially when it comes to the art of healing. If the rest of the physicians and herbalists have healed what you heal, they too would be more arrogant.

Q.- What? They are arrogant?

H.- Arrogant is a demonstration of being self-confident. We don't see that among our people. So, when we do see it among our people, the people of color. Even people of color will react to that as that person is arrogant. Because they are conditioned too.

Q.- I want to get back to some basic ailments that some of our people are confronted with right now. Young brothers are showing up with kidney ailments. What would you attribute kidney ailment to at a young age? Also, young sisters having thyroid tumor and reproductive problems in their 20's, something that should show up later. Would you say that it started from... the colon?

H.- No! It doesn't start in the colon. I used to say that too, that every disease begins in the colon. But if that was true... What habits are putting the things that are going to the colon that makes us sick? Why are we eating the things that enter the colon that make us sick? It is before the colon. It starts here in our brain.

Q.- It's in the mind.

H.- Not the mind, I don't know what the mind is. I have never found the mind. I hear people talk about the mind. I don't know what that is... but I do know this; when the brain is confused, you have problems. You would put anything in your mouth. Do you see this hand and this big mouth? Everything goes in there and it hasn't hit the colon yet. It starts in the brain. The brain has been confused. The computer has been confused. G in G out. Garbage in garbage out. But we don't want to see that. We want to rely on spirit, mind, and soul. When these are the prophets... What supernatural world do I live in? A natural world! In a natural world, there is no such thing as a mind. There is no such thing as a spirit or a soul.

Q.- You mentioned before about wanting to become spiritual and you went and met some of these people. And they had a stomach that can hardly fit through the door and you said this is spiritual? I don't think I want that.

H.- No! I don't subscribe to spirituality. Because all the spiritual people are big and fat and they have a problem with their head. So, I knew there was something I had to stay away from. I didn't pursue it any longer to see if there was any validity in this or not.

Q.- As far as our people and the New Age Movement are on course with the New Age Spiritual Movement. What is the relationship you would say then between the spirituality or say in the Motherland or the Native American or the Native Aborigine healers or witch doctors? Is there a science or is it fantasy or is there a combination? What's the reality in that?

H.- I don't know what it is. Because if it's so equitable among the Native Americans or the indigenous Indians as we call them. Why do they have the highest alcoholics among them? How come they can't even cure that? We got problems among the Africans too, they're eating garlic and hog. We have problems.

Spirituality is a word that comes out of Europe. Even the very word is European like the word "African." That's not African. That's not us, that's European. The continent was called Africa by them. There's a word they call spirituality. What is it? I don't know, not even interested.

Q.- If you were allowed to open a school. Where would you begin? Would you start with the plants?

H.- Oh...I gotta go way before the plants. I got to show you where we were derailed and change that environment. That brain environment. I have to change that immediately! Then you can begin to see. Because with the image that you're going to see, it is not the image that I would see. Because all of us are individually put together. We are unique, unlike the Athen. I would put together individually a package that

will unveil to him the privilege to see. And in seeing, then he can make the right decision, a good decision. My Grandmother started me out by understanding that I was not supposed to listen to anyone. No one! But yourself. And if I had to go outside of me. Train your eyes to watch Mother Nature in the forest.

Q.- Going back to these diseases and ailments. I know a lot of brothers and sisters and those who have passed on from AIDS. As a matter of fact, a brother from Bellevue Hospital. I went to go see him three days before he died from the so-called "Kaposi Sarcoma". He was getting chemotherapy and in his last days, he suffered. I want to ask you is there a way we can halt the progression and eliminate the ailments? With any disease AIDS, cancer, and so on.

H.- That's all we have been doing for the last 20 years.

Q.- To restore the body to normal.

H.- That's the only way to cure. That's the cure! To remove that particular erosion. To remove that particular condition. Whatever condition whether it's AIDS or blindness. We restore 100% health. That's the only way I can do it. Through what? Intra Cellular Cleansing. This is what is done in Miami. We put together compounds based on an electric system. Where do you go to America or New York and find electric food in a bottle? Where do you go? We only have to ask that one question. Is the body electrical? Yes! So, therefore it necessitates electric food. Where would you find that in New York?

Q.- AIDS is spreading rapidly. This so-called AIDS epidemic. I find the lesser disease is virtually being ignored such as herpes, lupus, sickle cell anemia, diabetes, specifically the sexually transmitted diseases.

H.- You ask about sexually transmitted diseases? Those are not lesser. There's only one disease. There have never been two diseases in the world. There's only been one disease. The compromise of the mucus membrane. The mucus membrane of the African has been compromised for 500 years now. What has the African ate since he left Africa? That is equable to his system? He has not eaten anything that will serve him equitably.

His biological structure has been weakening for over a period of 500 years. And in weakening the biological structure, then you may get lupus and herpes. You may get anything because the body has been deprived. The immune system has been compromised and the immune system is responsible for diabetes, leukemia, sickle cell for every disease in the world. Including that! Don't only attribute AIDS to the immune system. If your immune system is strong. You cannot get sick with any disease. We are going to straighten that.

Q.- What is the relation between medical science that's been around for 265 years with the laboratory reports and the blood break down. Is there any validity or goodness out of the allopathic medicine through the microscope and the relation of the electric foods?

H.- If you want to see a germ, you'll need a microscope. If you have a wound from a gunshot

or an appendix has burst, you need to be opened real quick. So, there's space for the knife but only in extreme conditions. But as far as curing diseases, there's only one way. That is the herbs. Because they are electrical. The molecular structure is complete. They will assimilate. Because they are carbon-based.

Q.- That's why in Egypt they had scaffold and knives, but what were the food of Egypt the Ptolemaic civilization.

H.- Ptolemaic people were hybrid, weren't they? Don't get angry. Be for real, stand up! That's why Cleopatra had to go all the way to Italy to find a man. She couldn't marry some Black man. She could not do that because she wasn't Black. She was a mixture of Persian, Greek, and Black. That's a hybrid person. So, the Egyptians ate hybrid food. Then they eat duck. One day they decide to make up garlic. What could Egyptians eat and didn't?

Opus, one of the first physicians that were given credit, an attribute to the first doctor. Did he open a human body? Yes, he did. He opened a human body. If the human body was meant to be opened, it would have a zipper.

Q.- There's another medical issue that I like to bring up. A big concern in this country is paralysis. How does the process of curing somebody with paralysis go, as far as your concern?

H.- The African Biomineral Balance had addressed that many years ago many, many times. In Salvadore, my friend Mr. Herbon Sanders fell off a log. He was in a wheelchair for 18 years. He's walking now.

Zadia Zeufi from New York from the University of Cornell. She came to us and she was in a wheelchair for 18 years. She's walking now. And many, many, many more!

Paralysis is what? When the central nervous system won't allow the muscle to contract or the nervous system is not sending enough electricity to make them move. So, what do we do? We perform again the Intra Cellular Cleansing and apply the African Biomineral Balance to regenerate the body with electricity and that could only be done the African way.

Q.- I want to ask you, my eyes used to be 20/20. How can I get it back to that?

H.- Well, I had an experience in Chicago with my own eyes. I didn't have any problems with my eyes, but I thought... I could read. I could see clearly. But then one day. I decided to do urine therapy. I use my compound for 20 days. I fast for a month, about 29 days. After my urine was clear like water, I decided to drink it. I was drinking it twice a day along with a gallon of water. At the end of the 4th day, I was completely blind. Completely blind! I was blind that Thursday, Friday, Saturday, Sunday, Monday. I began to see on Tuesday. I bought some blinder. I told my daughter to buy me some blinder.

"Please, quick! Because the sun was coming and it's hurting me."

She went and she got some blinders and I put them over my eyes. Oh, I was in darkness for five days. At the ending of the fifth day on my sixth day. I was in Chicago. I was on Coney Island where we had a center. When I took the blinders off. I could read the finest letter across the street.

So why was I blind? It was breaking all of the inflammation from my head down across my eyes. As it crosses the eyes, I had to go blind! You see, so what you need is a total fast for a while and do the therapy. Then you continue to diet and your eyes are going to come back immediately clear.

Q.- What happened to Dr. Clark?

H.- Dr. Clark, well you know.

Q.- Is it too late for him?

H.- It's not too late for anyone. But how much is he indebted to his Mother and Father? Dr. Clark is a beautiful brother. Dr. Clark needed help and he came to me.

I said "Dr. Clark, you can't eat these things"

And I love Dr. Clark. All of us do. Who doesn't? But Dr. Clark can't stop eating those things. Dr. Clark is like the brother by the name of Chancellor Williams. I went to see Chancellor Williams.

I said "My daughter is dying to meet you because you wrote the book "The Destruction of the Black Civilization."

In my house my children don't read books, none of them. Including myself. I don't read books. I just don't, never have, and never will. But that doesn't mean that books are bad.

Alright, but my daughter has read your book. She's happy to know that you're alive and she's happy to know today we're here to help you. Because you're going blind. Mr. Williams told me that he was OK. Dr. Coin told him that he was OK. He believes more in the Caucasian than he believes in his brother. So, we just went home.

Q.- Can you talk about sickle cell?

H.- Sickle cell anemia?

Q.- Yes, what's happening in the body and the effect of your tonic?

H.- Well, when I'm asked about sickle cell anemia. My brain goes to one country and that country is Ivory Coast. In Ivory Coast, 33% of the population has a high incidence of sickle cell anemia. 33%! I talked to Dr. Landenberg, he's a freshman about sickle cell anemia at Howard University. He disregards me. "But I cured sickle cell anemia," I told him.

I asked him, "What is sickle cell anemia?"

He said, "I don't know."

I said, "I thought so."

Because sickle cell anemia is when blood plasma has broken down by what? Mucus has seeped into the plasma. Into the cells themselves and break it and

disunite the cells. To unite the cells and to maintain that level. You have to feed the patient a large dose of iron phosphate, not ferrous oxide. Iron phosphate!

I don't know anyone in America that says that! But the sickle cell is when the same mucus that breaks down the cells in your nasal passage is called sinusitis. Has now broken down the blood plasma and breaks it into a sickle. Now, we have to replace the minerals that have been lost. Because iron phosphate incidentally is the only magnetic mineral on the planet. Being magnetic it pulls other minerals to it. So, when you take iron and you take all the other in proportionate balance. You'll see results in less than 5 minutes.

Q.- Malt liquor, what damage is that doing to the body? What is it doing to the mind when you consume it?

H.- The liver is damaged. Malt liquor is made out of what? Barley and I know they use the substance known as yeast. And isn't yeast a seed for infection? They call it what? Chlamydia. Yeast is the bed for the disease. But again, since we have not had scientists or researchers as they're called. To come forth with the proper research or studies. We fall short. We're vulnerable.

We are vulnerable. I just came to New York 10 years ago and they were drinking carrot juice. Carrot juice?! Well, that tells me something. They're eating beans in the name of health. That tells me that something is wrong. So, therefore we have to stop it.

The brother that came from DC said "There was a war on AIDS." And I was taken to Manhattan. War on AIDS?! I went to Dr. Barbara Jenson and Dr. Prince and they disregarded me.

And then said, "Dr. Alim is coming from Washington."

They said "A Muslim brother."

I said "A Muslim brother?"

They said, "Yes, He's coming with a very special message."

I said, "Yes, what is he coming to tell us?"

"AIDS kills black people."

I said, "We need to hear that from Dr. Alim?"

Because we were totally oblivious to that fact... But the question I'm going to ask about Dr. Alim, Is he a Muslim?

They said "Yes."

What is a Muslim that follows Allah doing practicing the medicine of the bliss, they call the devil? There is a contradiction.

Q.- What can WE do to keep your message alive to get your message across to all people?

H.- When the Japanese scientist said he worked with the immune system, all of Japan got behind him. He didn't ask them. They got behind him and he got the Nobel Peace Prize for only working with the immune system. We don't work with the immune system. When the Jews from Israel needed help. They didn't come asking for help from us. They sent help. So, you ask me "What could I say to help Usha research?" I don't know. If they help me, fine. If they don't help me, still fine. I don't know. That's on you. That's on the black populace. Not on us, we did our job.

Q.- Can you explain how cancer works in the body.

H.- The same way a common cold starts. In any part of the body, anywhere where cancer appears. It means that there's a condition that has manifested over and above. It's been progressively getting worse unattended or unknowing. There's no difference between cancer and the common cold. The mucus in the nose stays a long time, they call it sinusitis. And it begins to eat the cells, they call it cancer. That can be in the reproductive organs, the breasts, the head, the brain, the eyes, or wherever. It's all mucus.

Q.- You heard of Dr. Tory from Chicago? He teaches about the worms in the body. How they got there. What are zits made of? He said the worm doo-doo in your body and that's why you get zits.

H.- I disagree with that. When you open a zit. Inside of it, all you find is calcium carbonate. That's all you find. I can't challenge anyone or anything. But I do know this - that Dr. Tory has a compound that I know comes from the Caucasian's book. Larry White from Los Angeles, California. That's who groomed him, the White boy groomed him.

Q.- So in other words it is protection?

H.- What's the protection?

Q.- The zit, because you said it has carbon in it.

H.- No, calcium carbonate hardens. The mucus had hardened. Now it is growing and then it's going to burst and eat you up.

Q.- What is the effect of your tonic?

H.- My tonic, the Usha tonic electric food. Did you see Usha research, when the lady passed the tumor? It was in the refrigerator. She brought it in a bottle and we put it in the freezer. Tumor size of a silver dollar.

Q.- How did it come out?

H.- The only way it would come out.

Q.- It's supposed to come out through the regular holes, nose, mouth, or anus?

H.- Like Torus Henderson 1990. She had a tumor in her brain. This was recorded on channel 21 and channel 19 in Chicago by brother Raychem. She passed the tumor through the nose from her brain. Not only here. This Caucasian male, his daughter named Robin Bennett called me and said "My father has a tumor in his brain. A blood clot in his brain."

I said "Yes"

"How long will it take for you to take it out?"

I said, "How long have you allowed me?"

she said, "I give you a month."

I said, "How about 24 hours."

she said, "You're crazy."

Of course. It comes out in 24 hours and she wrote me a letter and I have that letter.

Q.- Do more Black people come to you? In terms of Honduras, who are the folks who are coming to you?

H.- Mexicans, Norwegian, South African, Whites. I don't expect Blacks from Africa to come. Chileans, Columbia, Americans, Latin America, Black America. Black America is down there now, with our most beloved professor John Simmon. But the general population at the Usha are Latinos and Europeans.

Q.- Can you please give some parting words to the world that will lead them to live a healthy life?

H.- My parting words would be this. Make sure that whenever you put something in your mouth, that something is going to compliment you and it's going to serve you well. It's going to support your nervous system. Because if you don't, you'll find yourself stressed. Not only are you going to find reasons to dislike me. You're going to dislike yourself. Glucose is the greatest enemy you will ever be faced with. Avoid it, because the one thing that you want to do is to love and that love should begin with you. Once you love you. You'll love the whole world. It's easy, it's delicious to love everybody and everything.

GOD's Recommended Medicine

Arnica (Arnica montana, Radix Ptarmicae Montanae, arnica flowers, mountain tobacco) is a powerful anti-inflammatory and antiseptic herb. It is used primarily to treat external wounds, and it relieves pain and promotes tissue regeneration. Arnica is used externally in the form of creams and compresses to treat arthritis, sprains, bruises, and headaches. Arnica infusions are used for their antiseptic properties to clean wounds, abscesses, and boils.

Batana oil (*Elaeis oleifera, American oil palm, palm oil*) is made from the kernel of the fruit of the Elaeis oleifera tree. The oil is used primarily for its fatty acids, nutrients, and phytonutrients as a hair oil to strengthen hair, to promote its growth, and as a natural hair coloring. It naturally turns gray hair brown.

Bladderwrack (*Fucus vesiculosus, fucus*) is used primarily because it is a high source of iodine. Bladderwrack has been used traditionally to treat an underactive and oversized thyroid and to treat iodine deficiency. Bladderwrack is also rich in calcium, magnesium, and potassium, and it contains other trace minerals. Bladderwrack contains numerous phytonutrients, which are credited with its many health benefits. Fucoxanthin anchors its antioxidant benefits. Bladderwrack has antiestrogenic effects and has been shown to lower the risk of estrogen-dependent diseases. Bladderwrack lowers lipid and cholesterol levels and supports weight loss. Its mucopolysaccharide phytonutrients inhibit skin enzymes from breaking down in the skin, reduce skin thickness, and improve elasticity. Bladderwrack has also shown anticandida, antibacterial, and antitumor properties.

Blessed thistle (*Cnicus benedictus, cardo santo, centaurea benedicta, folia cardui benedicti, holy thistle*) belongs to the Asteraceae plant family. Blessed thistle is high in iron and has been used in traditional medicine to increase circulation and oxygen delivery to the brain, to support brain function, and to support heart and lung function. Its bitter phytonutrients are used to support liver and gallbladder function and to stimulate the upper digestive tract to promote proper digestion and improve appetite.

Blessed thistle has antifungal and diuretic properties and has been used traditionally for its emmenagogue properties that treat hormonal disorders that interfere with normal menstruation. Blessed thistle is also considered a galactagogue and has been used to increase and enrich milk flow in nursing mothers. Blessed thistle is also used to remove toxins, acids, and mucus and to assist in intracellular cleansing (inside cells).

Blue vervain (*Verbena hastate, simpler's joy, verbena*) has diuretic, antimalarial, anti-inflammatory, and antimicrobial properties. Blue vervain has been used in traditional medicine as a female tonic to treat menstrual cramps and as an emmenagogue to increase milk production in women who are breastfeeding. The Primary use of blue vervain is to treat nervous disorders including, stress, anxiety, and restlessness.

Burdock Root (*Arctium lappa*) is also known as bardana. Burdock root is a diuretic, blood cleanser, anti-inflammatory, antioxidant, antifungal, anticancer, antiviral, and antibacterial herb. Many chemical compounds, which include inulin, mucilage, essential oil, volatile oil, alkaloids, glycosides, resin, and tannins. Burdock has been used in traditional medicine to treat skin conditions such as eczema, acne, and psoriasis because it promotes the removal of toxins from the skin. It is also a diuretic used to promote urination to stimulate kidney function and repair. The primary use of burdock root is as a blood purifier and liver tonic to restore liver function and health.

Cascara Sagrada (*Rhamnus purshiana, sacred bark, pushiana, purschiana bark, persiana bark, chittam bark*) contains emodin, which has antiviral and anticancer properties. Cascara sagrada is used primarily as a laxative and stimulates the peristaltic action of the intestine. This wavelike motion moves waste through the intestine. This property helps restore the proper tone and health of the intestine by pushing waste out of diverticula pouches that develop in the intestinal wall. This helps restore the mucous lining and health of the intestine. Cascara sagrada has been used in traditional medicine to improve stomach, liver, and pancreas secretions and to break up and remove gallstones from the gallbladder.

Chaparral (*Larrea tridentate, gobernadora*) has antimicrobial and antibacterial, antitumor and anticancer, and antiulcerogenic and anti-inflammatory properties. Traditionally, chaparral has been used to kill parasites; address sexually transmitted diseases; treat skin conditions like eczema, psoriasis, skin rashes, and bruises; and as an expectorant to treat respiratory issues like colds and bronchitis.

Cocolmeca (*Smilax, Smilax regelii, Smilax aristolochiifolia, Jamaican sarsaparilla cocomeca bark, cuculmeca*) has anti-inflammatory, antiulcer, antioxidant, anticancer, diaphoretic, and diuretic properties. Cocolmeca is a plant of the Smilax genus and has been shown to bind with toxins for their removal from the blood and body. Cocolmeca is used in traditional medicine to treat skin conditions like psoriasis and leprosy, rheumatoid arthritis and joint pain, headaches, colds, and sexual impotence.

Contribo (*Aristolochia, Aristolochia grandiflora, Birthwort, duck flower, Alcatraz, hierba del Indio*) is used in traditional medicine for arthritis and edema, to stimulate the immune system and white-blood-cell production, to kill parasites, and to treat snakebites.

Damiana (*Turnera diffusa, turnera, turnea aprodisiaca, damiana aphrodisiaca, damiana herb, damiana leaf*) has anti-aromatase and antianxiety properties. Men and women use damiana to strengthen the sexual organs and boost sexual drive and potency. The anti-aromatase property blocks androstenedione and estrogen related illness in women like breast cancer and fibroids. Women also use it to reduce hot flashes associated with menopause.

It also helps balance estrogen and supports testosterone levels in men. Damiana increases oxygen delivery to the genitals, resulting in increased libido. Damiana is also used to treat depression and nervousness and to relieve anxiety associated with sexual dysfunction. Damiana stimulates the intestinal tract and is used to treat constipation.

Elderberry (*Sambucus, Sambucus nigra, Sambucus africana*) has anti-inflammatory, antiviral, anti-influenza, and anticancer properties. It is used to treat colds, the flu, and allergies and to remove mucus from the respiratory system. Sambucus nigra is most commonly used medicinally because it has been shown to be non-toxic, while other species can be toxic. Sambucus nigra has been shown in studies to bind with the H1N1 virus and stop it from entering cells.

Eyebright (*Euphrasia Officinalis, Euphrasia rostkoviana*) has anti-inflammatory and antiseptic properties and is used as an eyewash to soothe the eye's mucous membrane and to treat chronic inflammation of the eye. Eyebright is used as an antimicrobial to treat conjunctivitis and blepharitis bacterial infection of the eye. Eyebright is used as an astringent to treat wounds and reduce skin inflammation. It is also used internally as an anti-inflammatory to treat upper respiratory infections like sinusitis and hay fever.

Guaco (*Mikania guaco, Mikania glomerata, guace, bejuco de Finca, cepu, liane Francois, matafinca, vedolin, cipo caatinga, huaco, erva das Serpentes*) has anti-inflammatory, antiallergic, and bronchodilator properties. Guaco is used primarily in traditional medicine for upper respiratory problems like asthma, bronchitis, colds, and flu. It is used as an anti-inflammatory agent for rheumatoid arthritis and inflammation in the digestive tract and as an antibacterial for Candida and yeast infections. Guaco contains around 10 percent coumarin, which has blood-thinning properties.

Huereque (*Ibervillea sonorae, guareque, wareki, choyalhuani, wereke, big root, coyote melon, cowpie plant*) has hypoglycemic, antiobesity, and antimicrobial properties. Huereque is used in traditional medicine to lower blood sugar levels, treat diabetes, and reduce weight. It is used to nourish and cleanse the pancreas.

Hombre grande (*Picrasma excelsa, Quassia amara L., quassia, cuassia mara, Jamaican quassia, Amargo, bitter ash, bitter bark, bitter wood*) has antifungal, antiulcer, antimalarial, anticancer, and insecticide properties. Hombre grande has been used in traditional medicine topically to treat measles and orally to treat constipation and diarrhea, intestinal parasite infections, and fever. It is used to stimulate the digestive tract and bile production, increase appetite, cleanse the blood, and stimulate enzyme production. Hombre grande helps rebalance the flora in the digestive tract to support the immune system.

Hops (*Humulus lupulus, lupulo*) has antibacterial, anti-inflammatory, and anticancer properties. Hops are used in traditional medicine to break up inflammation; relieve pain; promote digestion, urination, and appetite; treat rheumatic pains, infections, insomnia, and sleeping disorders; and anxiety, tension, attention deficit hyperactivity disorder (ADHD), irritability, and nervousness.

Hydrangea Root (*Hydrangea, Hydrangea arborescens, hortensia, seven barks*) has anti-inflammatory, lithotrophic, antiseptic, antiparasitic, and autoimmune properties. Hydrangea is used for its hydrating compound, which dissolves calcium deposits in soft tissue. It has been used traditionally to treat bladder and kidney disease, to dissolve kidney stones, and to clean the lymphatic system. Chang Shan is used in Chinese medicine for its febrifuge compound to treat autoimmune diseases.

Lavender (*Lavandula*) has antifungal, antibacterial, analgesic, anti-inflammatory, anti-insomnia, anticonvulsant, antispasmodic, and antianxiety and antidepressant properties. Lavender is used as a traditional medicine to treat restlessness, insomnia, nervousness, and depression. Lavender is used for migraines, nerve pain, and joint pain. It is also used to reverse abdominal swelling from gas, upset stomach, nausea, loss of appetite, and vomiting.

Lily of the Valley (*Convallaria majalis, clochette des Bois, constancy, convallaria, convallaria herba, convall-lily, gazon de Parnassus, Jacob's ladder, ladder-to-heaven, our lady's tears*) has antiangiogenic, antitumor, and diuretic properties. Lily of the valley has been used for hundreds of years in traditional medicine primarily as a heart tonic to treat heart failure and irregular heartbeat. Lily of the valley's action is similar to the drug Digitalis, but it is natural, less concentrated, and therefore less powerful. It is used to treat heart debility and dropsy. It promotes increased oxygen delivery to the heart, reduces blood pressure, and relaxes a weak heart to beat more slowly and efficiently while increasing its power.

Mullein (*Verbascum, Verbascum thapsus, Aaron's rod, Indian tobacco, Jacob's staff, Peter's staff, blanket leaf, Bullock's lungwort, cow's lungwort, feltwort, hare's beard, lady's foxglove, mullein leaf*) has antiparasitic and antispasmodic, antibacterial, antiviral, anti-inflammatory, antitubercular, and anti-influenza properties. Mullein is used primarily as an expectorant to remove mucus from the respiratory tract, including the lungs.

Nettle (*Urtica dioica, ortiga, stinging nettle*) has anti-inflammatory, anticancer, diuretic, antioxidant, antimicrobial, antiulcer, and analgesic activities. Nettle root is used for an enlarged prostate, for joints, and as a diuretic and astringent. Nettle leaves are used for arthritis, sore muscles, hair loss, anemia, poor circulation, diabetes, enlarged spleen, allergies, eczema and rash, and asthma. Nettle is used as a general health tonic and blood purifier.

Nopal (*Opuntia, Prickly pear, nopal cactus*) is the paddle of the Opuntia cactus, which also produces the prickly-pear fruit. Nopal contains numerous phytochemicals, antioxidants, vitamins, and minerals. It is used to reverse type 2 diabetes, high cholesterol, obesity, alcohol hangover, colitis, diarrhea, and viral infections.

Prodigiosa (*Brickellia canvanillesi, prodigiosa, amula, hamula, calea zacatechichi, dream herb, cheech, bitter grass*) is used in traditional medicine to stimulate pancreas and liver secretions, increasing bile synthesis and evacuation of bile from the gallbladder. Prodigiosa is used to treat diabetes by controlling blood sugar levels. Prodigiosa is used to treat headaches and fever. Prodigiosa has anti-anxiety properties and induces a vivid dream state.

Red Clover (*Trifolium pratense, meadow honeysuckle, meadow trefoil, purple clover, trefoil, wild clover, cleaver grass, marl grass, cow grass*) has anticancer, diuretic, expectorant, and sedative, anti-inflammatory, and anti-atherosclerosis properties. Red clover is used for its estrogen properties to relieve menopausal symptoms. Red clover is a blood purifier and is used to break up calcification in soft tissues and to clean the lymphatic system of lymph fluid waste.

Rhubarb Root (*Rheum palmatum, Chinese rhubarb, Turkish rhubarb, Indian rhubarb, Russian rhubarb, R. tanguticum, and R. officinale - dahuang*) has antioxidant, heavy-metal chelation, anticancer, and antibacterial properties. Rhubarb root is used to regulate the digestive tract to treat digestive issues that include diarrhea, constipation, stomach pain, and acid reflux. Rhubarb root hemorrhoids and tears of the lining of the anus. Rhubarb root is used to treat kidney stones and kidney disease, to chelate heavy metals, to remove acids and mucus, and to intracellularly cleanse cells.

Sage (*Salvia officinalis*) has antioxidant, antimicrobial, anti-inflammatory, antitumor, antidiarrheal, and anti-obesity properties. Sage has also been shown to reduce LDL cholesterol and raise HDL cholesterol, improving the HDL/LDL ratio. Sage is used in traditional medicine to improve memory, treat menopausal hot flashes, reduce gastrointestinal inflammation, nourish the pancreas, and treat diabetes.

Santa Maria (*Tagetes lucida, pericon, hierbanis, yerbanis, Mexican marigold, Mexican tarragon*) has antifungal and antibacterial, antidepressant, antioxidant and analgesic, and anti-inflammatory properties. Santa Maria is used in traditional medicine to treat diarrhea, abdominal pains, respiratory infections, rheumatism, and inflammatory skin diseases. Santa Maria has psychoactive properties and is used to relax the nerves.

Sapo (*Eryngium carlinae, yerba del Sapo, hierba del Sapo, grass frog, grass toad*) has hypolipidemic, antioxidant, and anti-inflammatory properties. Sapo is used in traditional medicine to lower cholesterol and triglyceride levels in the blood and arteries. Sapo is used to treat gallstones and kidney stones.

Sarsaparilla (*Smilax, Hemidesmus indicus*) can refer to two species of plant, Smilax or Hemidesmus indicus. Smilax comes from South America, and Hemidesmus indicus comes from India, and they have similar properties. They have anti-inflammatory, antiulcer, antioxidant, anticancer, diaphoretic, and diuretic properties. Sarsaparilla has been shown to bind with toxins for their removal from the blood and body. Sarsaparilla is used in traditional medicine to treat skin conditions like psoriasis and leprosy, rheumatoid arthritis and joint pain, headaches, colds, and sexual impotence.

Sea Moss (*Chondrus crispus, Irish moss*) has antibacterial, anti-inflammatory, and laxative properties. Sea moss is used for its demulcent properties to soothe irritated mucous membranes from colds, coughs, bronchitis, tuberculosis, gastric ulcers, and intestinal problems. Sea moss is used to support joint and skin health, and its wide range of nutrients serve as a natural mineral supplement.

Sensitiva (*Mimosa sensitiva, Mimosa pudica*) has antidepressant, anticonvulsant, antibacterial, diuretic, antioxidant, anti-inflammatory, and aphrodisiac properties. Sensitiva is used in traditional medicine to relieve hemorrhoid and arthritis pain, stop bleeding, and treat uterine infections. Sensitiva is also used to increase sexual desire and libido.

Shea Butter (*Vitellaria paradoxa, Butyrospermum paradoxa, Butyrospermum parkii*) is the nut is the shea tree Vitellaria paradoxa and is traditional African plant food. It is popularly used for skin treatment. Shea butter made from the shea nut is rich in skin-protective fatty acids, nutrients, and phytonutrients. It is used to moisturize the skin, increase elasticity, and treat conditions like blemishes, wrinkles, sunburn, eczema, and small wounds.

Tila (*Tilia, linden, basswood*) has antioxidant, neuroprotective, anticonvulsant and antiseizure, antispasmodic, anti-inflammatory, anticancer, and diuretic properties. Linden is used in traditional medicine to support the immune system, relax nerves, relieve depression, and treat insomnia, fever, headaches, migraines, inflammatory skin conditions, and the liver and gallbladder.

Urtila Oil (*Urtila dioica, Urtica dioica*) extracted from the nettle plant is used as a hair conditioner and to support oil production in the scalp.

Valerian (*Valerianu officinalis L Veleriana, valerian, capon's tail, all-heal, garden heliotrope, English valerian, Vermont valeria, setwall, wild valerian*) has sedative, anticonvulsant, antianxiety, and antidepressant properties. It relieves anxiety, nervousness, exhaustion, headache, and hysteria. Valerian is used to relaxing and strengthening the uterus.

Yellow Dock Root (*Rumex crispus, curly dock*) has antioxidant, antimicrobial, antibacterial, anti-inflammatory, and analgesic and antipyretic properties. Yellow dock stimulates bile production, aiding in the digestion of fat, and stimulates bowel movement to clear the digestive tract. Yellow dock has been used in traditional medicine as a blood purifier and liver and gallbladder cleanser and to clean the lymphatic system.

Yohimbe (*Corvanthe yohimbe, Pausinystalia johimbe, yohimbe bark, yohimbine*) has antiobesity, antidepressant, and libido-enhancing properties. Yohimbe is used in traditional medicine to increase sexual desire and to reverse erectile impotence. Though Yohimbe is used more often for male libido, it is also effective in increasing female sexual desire and performance.

GOD's Creations

Vegetables: Amaranth greens, Wild Arugula, Avocado, Bell Peppers, Chayote (Mexican Squash), Cucumber, Dandelion Greens, Garbanzo Beans, Izote – cactus flower/cactus leaf, Kale, Lettuce (all, except Iceberg) Mushrooms (all, except Shitake), Nopales – Mexican Cactus, Okra, Olives, Onions, Sea Vegetables (wakame/dulse/arame/hijiki/nori), Squash, Tomato – cherry and plum only, Tomatillo, Turnip greens, Zucchini, Watercress, Purslane (Verdolaga).

Fruits: Apples, Bananas – the smallest one or the Burro/mid-size (original banana) Berries – all varieties-Elderberries in any form – no cranberries, Cantaloupe, Cherries, Currants, Dates, Figs, Grapes- seeded, Limes (key limes preferred with seeds), Mango, Melons- seeded, Orange (Seville or sour preferred, difficult to find), Papayas, Peaches, Pears, Plums, Prickly Pear (Cactus Fruit), Prunes, Raisins- seeded, Soft Jelly Coconuts, Soursops - (Latin or West Indian markets).

All-Natural Herbal Teas: Burdock, Chamomile, Elderberry, Fennel, Ginger, Raspberry, Tila.

Grains: Amaranth, Fonio, Kamut, Quinoa, Rye, Spelt, Tef, Wild Rice.

Nuts & Seeds (includes Nuts & Seed Butters): Hempseed, Raw Sesame Seeds, Raw Sesame "Tahini" Butter, Walnuts, Brazil Nuts.

Oils: Olive Oil (uncooked), Coconut Oil (uncooked), Grapeseed oil, Sesame Oil, Hemp Seed Oil, Avocado Oil.

Mild Flavors: Basil, Bay leaf, Cloves, Dill, Oregano, Savory, Sweet Basil, Tarragon, Thyme.

Pungent & Spicy Flavors: Achiote, Cayenne/African Bird Pepper, Onion Powder, Habanero, Sage

Salty Flavors: Pure Sea Salt, Powdered Granulated Seaweed (Kelp/Dulce/Nori - has "sea taste")

Sweet Flavors: Pure Agave Syrup (from cactus), Date Sugar

Acknowledgments

Alfredo "Dr. Sebi" Bowman

11/26/1933 - 8/6/2016

Thank you.

INDEX

A
Al Sharpton 51

B
Bell's Palsy 102

C
Chancellor Williams 116
Chemotherapy 68, 112
Chlamydia 118
Chondrus Crispus 70, 132
Cleopatra 11, 114
Common cold 84, 120

D
Dick Gregory 33, 34, 92
Dr. Victor Herbert 65

E
Elijah Mohammed 41, 58, 88
Eugenia Charles 73

F
Farrakhan 51
Ferrous Oxide 118

G
George Washington
Carver 54, 92

H
Hippocrates 44, 62, 67, 69, 84
Holy Bible 62

I
Intracellular Chelation 60
Iron phosphate 118

J
Jesse Jackson 51

K
Kaposi Sarema 112

L
Law of life 14, 29
Lisa "Left-Eye"
  Lopez 70

M
Marco Polo 90
Michael Jackson 11, 59

N
Nelson Mandela 73
New York Supreme
  Court 60

P
Paralysis 61, 114, 115
Ptolemaic 114

R
Retinitis Pigmentosa
  74, 76
Robert Abrams 61
Robert Mugabe 73

S
Sea Moss 28, 70, 132

U
Urine therapy 115

V
Vilcabamba 56

W
World Health
  Organization 97